Quick Overview

As you draw closer to taking your exam, effective preparation becomes more and more important. Thankfully, you have this study guide to help you get ready. Use this guide to help keep your studying on track and refer to it often.

This study guide contains several key sections that will help you be successful on your exam. The guide contains tips for what you should do the night before and the day of the test. Also included are test-taking tips. Knowing the right information is not always enough. Many well-prepared test takers struggle with exams. These tips will help equip you to accurately read, assess, and answer test questions.

A large part of the guide is devoted to showing you what content to expect on the exam and to helping you better understand that content. Near the end of this guide is a practice test so that you can see how well you have grasped the content. Then, answer explanations are provided so that you can understand why you missed certain questions.

Don't try to cram the night before you take your exam. This is not a wise strategy for a few reasons. First, your retention of the information will be low. Your time would be better used by reviewing information you already know rather than trying to learn a lot of new information. Second, you will likely become stressed as you try to gain a large amount of knowledge in a short amount of time. Third, you will be depriving yourself of sleep. So be sure to go to bed at a reasonable time the night before. Being well-rested helps you focus and remain calm.

Be sure to eat a substantial breakfast the morning of the exam. If you are taking the exam in the afternoon, be sure to have a good lunch as well. Being hungry is distracting and can make it difficult to focus. You have hopefully spent lots of time preparing for the exam. Don't let an empty stomach get in the way of success!

When travelling to the testing center, leave earlier than needed. That way, you have a buffer in case you experience any delays. This will help you remain calm and will keep you from missing your appointment time at the testing center.

Be sure to pace yourself during the exam. Don't try to rush through the exam. There is no need to risk performing poorly on the exam just so you can leave the testing center early. Allow yourself to use all of the allotted time if needed.

Remain positive while taking the exam even if you feel like you are performing poorly. Thinking about the content you should have mastered will not help you perform better on the exam.

Once the exam is complete, take some time to relax. Even if you feel that you need to take the exam again, you will be well served by some down time before you begin studying again. It's often easier to convince yourself to study if you know that it will come with a reward!

Test-Taking Strategies

1. Predicting the Answer

When you feel confident in your preparation for a multiple-choice test, try predicting the answer before reading the answer choices. This is especially useful on questions that test objective factual knowledge or that ask you to fill in a blank. By predicting the answer before reading the available choices, you eliminate the possibility that you will be distracted or led astray by an incorrect answer choice. You will feel more confident in your selection if you read the question, predict the answer, and then find your prediction among the answer choices. After using this strategy, be sure to still read all of the answer choices carefully and completely. If you feel unprepared, you should not attempt to predict the answers. This would be a waste of time and an opportunity for your mind to wander in the wrong direction.

2. Reading the Whole Question

Too often, test takers scan a multiple-choice question, recognize a few familiar words, and immediately jump to the answer choices. Test authors are aware of this common impatience, and they will sometimes prey upon it. For instance, a test author might subtly turn the question into a negative, or he or she might redirect the focus of the question right at the end. The only way to avoid falling into these traps is to read the entirety of the question carefully before reading the answer choices.

3. Looking for Wrong Answers

Long and complicated multiple-choice questions can be intimidating. One way to simplify a difficult multiple-choice question is to eliminate all of the answer choices that are clearly wrong. In most sets of answers, there will be at least one selection that can be dismissed right away. If the test is administered on paper, the test taker could draw a line through it to indicate that it may be ignored; otherwise, the test taker will have to perform this operation mentally or on scratch paper. In either case, once the obviously incorrect answers have been eliminated, the remaining choices may be considered. Sometimes identifying the clearly wrong answers will give the test taker some information about the correct answer. For instance, if one of the remaining answer choices is a direct opposite of one of the eliminated answer choices, it may well be the correct answer. The opposite of obviously wrong is obviously right! Of course, this is not always the case. Some answers are obviously incorrect simply because they are irrelevant to the question being asked. Still, identifying and eliminating some incorrect answer choices is a good way to simplify a multiple-choice question.

4. Don't Overanalyze

Anxious test takers often overanalyze questions. When you are nervous, your brain will often run wild, causing you to make associations and discover clues that don't actually exist. If you feel that this may be a problem for you, do whatever you can to slow down during the test. Try taking a deep breath or counting to ten. As you read and consider the question, restrict yourself to the particular words used by the author. Avoid thought tangents about what the author *really* meant, or what he or she was *trying* to say. The only things that matter on a multiple-choice test are the words that are actually in the question. You must avoid reading too much into a multiple-choice question, or supposing that the writer meant something other than what he or she wrote.

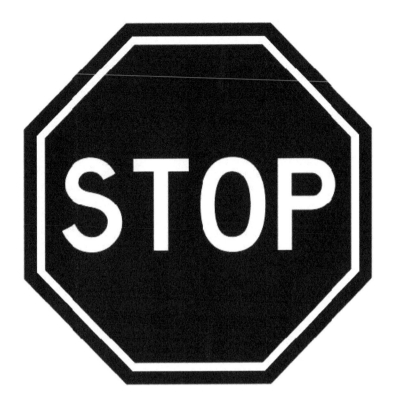

FREE Test Taking Tips DVD Offer

To help us better serve you, we have developed a Test Taking Tips DVD that we would like to give you for FREE. **This DVD covers world-class test taking tips that you can use to be even more successful when you are taking your test.**

All that we ask is that you email us your feedback about your study guide. Please let us know what you thought about it – whether that is good, bad or indifferent.

To get your **FREE Test Taking Tips DVD**, email freedvd@studyguideteam.com with "FREE DVD" in the subject line and the following information in the body of the email:

   a. The title of your study guide.

   b. Your product rating on a scale of 1-5, with 5 being the highest rating.

   c. Your feedback about the study guide. What did you think of it?

   d. Your full name and shipping address to send your free DVD.

If you have any questions or concerns, please don't hesitate to contact us at freedvd@studyguideteam.com.

Thanks again!

CMA Exam Preparation
Study Guide 2018-2019

Certified Medical Assistant Exam Preparation 2018 & 2019

Table of Contents

5. No Need for Panic

It is wise to learn as many strategies as possible before taking a multiple-choice test, but it is likely that you will come across a few questions for which you simply don't know the answer. In this situation, avoid panicking. Because most multiple-choice tests include dozens of questions, the relative value of a single wrong answer is small. Moreover, your failure on one question has no effect on your success elsewhere on the test. As much as possible, you should compartmentalize each question on a multiple-choice test. In other words, you should not allow your feelings about one question to affect your success on the others. When you find a question that you either don't understand or don't know how to answer, just take a deep breath and do your best. Read the entire question slowly and carefully. Try rephrasing the question a couple of different ways. Then, read all of the answer choices carefully. After eliminating obviously wrong answers, make a selection and move on to the next question.

6. Confusing Answer Choices

When working on a difficult multiple-choice question, there may be a tendency to focus on the answer choices that are the easiest to understand. Many people, whether consciously or not, gravitate to the answer choices that require the least concentration, knowledge, and memory. This is a mistake. When you come across an answer choice that is confusing, you should give it extra attention. A question might be confusing because you do not know the subject matter to which it refers. If this is the case, don't eliminate the answer before you have affirmatively settled on another. When you come across an answer choice of this type, set it aside as you look at the remaining choices. If you can confidently assert that one of the other choices is correct, you can leave the confusing answer aside. Otherwise, you will need to take a moment to try to better understand the confusing answer choice. Rephrasing is one way to tease out the sense of a confusing answer choice.

7. Your First Instinct

Many people struggle with multiple-choice tests because they overthink the questions. If you have studied sufficiently for the test, you should be prepared to trust your first instinct once you have carefully and completely read the question and all of the answer choices. There is a great deal of research suggesting that the mind can come to the correct conclusion very quickly once it has obtained all of the relevant information. At times, it may seem to you as if your intuition is working faster even than your reasoning mind. This may in fact be true. The knowledge you obtain while studying may be retrieved from your subconscious before you have a chance to work out the associations that support it. Verify your instinct by working out the reasons that it should be trusted.

8. Key Words

Many test takers struggle with multiple-choice questions because they have poor reading comprehension skills. Quickly reading and understanding a multiple-choice question requires a mixture of skill and experience. To help with this, try jotting down a few key words and phrases on a piece of scrap paper. Doing this concentrates the process of reading and forces the mind to weigh the relative importance of the question's parts. In selecting words and phrases to write down, the test taker thinks about the question more deeply and carefully. This is especially true for multiple-choice questions that are preceded by a long prompt.

9. Subtle Negatives

One of the oldest tricks in the multiple-choice test writer's book is to subtly reverse the meaning of a question with a word like *not* or *except*. If you are not paying attention to each word in the question, you can easily be led astray by this trick. For instance, a common question format is, "Which of the following is...?" Obviously, if the question instead is, "Which of the following is not...?," then the answer will be quite different. Even worse, the test makers are aware of the potential for this mistake and will include one answer choice that would be correct if the question were not negated or reversed. A test taker who misses the reversal will find what he or she believes to be a correct answer and will be so confident that he or she will fail to reread the question and discover the original error. The only way to avoid this is to practice a wide variety of multiple-choice questions and to pay close attention to each and every word.

10. Reading Every Answer Choice

It may seem obvious, but you should always read every one of the answer choices! Too many test takers fall into the habit of scanning the question and assuming that they understand the question because they recognize a few key words. From there, they pick the first answer choice that answers the question they believe they have read. Test takers who read all of the answer choices might discover that one of the latter answer choices is actually *more* correct. Moreover, reading all of the answer choices can remind you of facts related to the question that can help you arrive at the correct answer. Sometimes, a misstatement or incorrect detail in one of the latter answer choices will trigger your memory of the subject and will enable you to find the right answer. Failing to read all of the answer choices is like not reading all of the items on a restaurant menu: you might miss out on the perfect choice.

11. Spot the Hedges

One of the keys to success on multiple-choice tests is paying close attention to every word. This is never more true than with words like *almost*, *most*, *some*, and *sometimes*. These words are called "hedges" because they indicate that a statement is not totally true or not true in every place and time. An absolute statement will contain no hedges, but in many subjects, like literature and history, the answers are not always straightforward or absolute. There are always exceptions to the rules in these subjects. For this reason, you should favor those multiple-choice questions that contain hedging language. The presence of qualifying words indicates that the author is taking special care with his or her words, which is certainly important when composing the right answer. After all, there are many ways to be wrong, but there is only one way to be right! For this reason, it is wise to avoid answers that are absolute when taking a multiple-choice test. An absolute answer is one that says things are either all one way or all another. They often include words like *every*, *always*, *best*, and *never*. If you are taking a multiple-choice test in a subject that doesn't lend itself to absolute answers, be on your guard if you see any of these words.

12. Long Answers

In many subject areas, the answers are not simple. As already mentioned, the right answer often requires hedges. Another common feature of the answers to a complex or subjective question are qualifying clauses, which are groups of words that subtly modify the meaning of the sentence. If the question or answer choice describes a rule to which there are exceptions or the subject matter is complicated, ambiguous, or confusing, the correct answer will require many words in order to be expressed clearly and accurately. In essence, you should not be deterred by answer choices that seem excessively long. Oftentimes, the author of the text will not be able to write the correct answer without offering some qualifications and modifications. Your job is to read the answer choices thoroughly and completely and to select the one that most accurately and precisely answers the question.

13. Restating to Understand

Sometimes, a question on a multiple-choice test is difficult not because of what it asks but because of how it is written. If this is the case, restate the question or answer choice in different words. This process serves a couple of important purposes. First, it forces you to concentrate on the core of the question. In order to rephrase the question accurately, you have to understand it well. Rephrasing the question will concentrate your mind on the key words and ideas. Second, it will present the information to your mind in a fresh way. This process may trigger your memory and render some useful scrap of information picked up while studying.

14. True Statements

Sometimes an answer choice will be true in itself, but it does not answer the question. This is one of the main reasons why it is essential to read the question carefully and completely before proceeding to the answer choices. Too often, test takers skip ahead to the answer choices and look for true statements. Having found one of these, they are content to select it without reference to the question above. Obviously, this provides an easy way for test makers to play tricks. The savvy test taker will always read the entire question before turning to the answer choices. Then, having settled on a correct answer choice, he or she will refer to the original question and ensure that the selected answer is relevant. The mistake of choosing a correct-but-irrelevant answer choice is especially common on questions related to specific pieces of objective knowledge, like historical or scientific facts. A prepared test taker will have a wealth of factual knowledge at his or her disposal, and should not be careless in its application.

15. No Patterns

One of the more dangerous ideas that circulates about multiple-choice tests is that the correct answers tend to fall into patterns. These erroneous ideas range from a belief that B and C are the most common right answers, to the idea that an unprepared test-taker should answer "A-B-A-C-A-D-A-B-A." It cannot be emphasized enough that pattern-seeking of this type is exactly the WRONG way to approach a multiple-choice test. To begin with, it is highly unlikely that the test maker will plot the correct answers according to some predetermined pattern. The questions are scrambled and delivered in a random order. Furthermore, even if the test maker was following a pattern in the assignation of correct answers, there is no reason why the test taker would know which pattern he or she was using. Any attempt to discern a pattern in the answer choices is a waste of time and a distraction from the real work of taking the test. A test taker would be much better served by extra preparation before the test than by reliance on a pattern in the answers.

FREE DVD OFFER

Don't forget that doing well on your exam includes both understanding the test content and understanding how to use what you know to do well on the test. We offer a completely FREE Test Taking Tips DVD that covers world class test taking tips that you can use to be even more successful when you are taking your test.

All that we ask is that you email us your feedback about your study guide. To get your **FREE Test Taking Tips DVD**, email freedvd@studyguideteam.com with "FREE DVD" in the subject line and the following information in the body of the email:

- The title of your study guide.
- Your product rating on a scale of 1-5, with 5 being the highest rating.
- Your feedback about the study guide. What did you think of it?
- Your full name and shipping address to send your free DVD.

Introduction to the CMA Exam

Function of the Test

The Certified Medical Assistant (CMA) Exam is offered by the Certifying Board of the American Association of Medical Assistants (AAMA) as part of their program for credentialing medical assistants. Individuals taking the CMA Exam fall into one of three categories: 1) prospective or recent graduates of accredited medical assisting programs; 2) graduates applying more than twelve months after graduating from an accredited medical assisting program; or 3) candidates who previously passed the exam and are seeking recertification. Scores are generally used only for the certification process.

The exam is intended to impartially, objectively, and fairly measure a thorough, broad, and current understanding of health care delivery. It is taken by individuals seeking certification or recertification as medical assistants nationwide. In 2015, 17,324 individuals sought initial CMA Certification. Of that cohort, 10,573 test takers passed, yielding a 62% pass rate.

Test Administration

Individuals wishing to take the exam must apply through the AAMA. In the application, the individual must select their preferred 90-day testing window. If the application is approved, the individual must contact Prometric – the testing center that administers the exam. The individual must then select a test date, time, and location, and complete the exam within the assigned window.

Upon arrival at the test center, the test taker must furnish the appropriate identification. The test center will offer test takers lockers for personal items and then set each test taker up at a computer. Test takers are offered an optional tutorial to familiarize themselves with the test taking software. The tutorial lasts a maximum of fifteen minutes.

Individuals seeking certification for the first time are allowed three attempts to pass the exam. In accordance with the Americans with Disabilities Act, test takers with documented disabilities may request accommodations by submitting a Request for Special Accommodations form, which is available from the AAMA.

Test Format

The CMA Exam consists of 200 questions, 180 of which are scored and 20 of which are pretest questions. The pretest questions are included for evaluation of potential questions for future exams and are not scored, but the test taker is not informed as to which of the 200 total questions are pretest questions. The test is administered in four sessions of 40 minutes each; the total examination time is 2 hours and 40 minutes. Test takers may also take up to 20 minutes as break time between sections if they so choose.

The content of the exam falls into three major categories: General, Administrative, and Clinical. Within those categories, test takers receive questions on a wide variety of topics such as medical terminology, anatomy, physiology, and record keeping. The questions from the various categories are interspersed amongst each other throughout the exam.

Section	Category	# of Qs	Percent of Exam
1	General	50	28%
2	Administrative	45	25%
3	Clinical	85	47%
Total		**180**	**100%**
Unscored		**20**	**NA**

Scoring

Scores are based on the total number of correct answers provided by the test taker, with no penalty for wrong answers beyond the missed opportunity to get another answer correct. This raw score is standardized and converted to a scaled score. The Certifying Board sets the passing score at a level that indicates the minimum competency for an entry level medical assistant and adjusts it as appropriate. The current minimum passing score is 430.

The test taker receives an immediate pass/fail notification upon completion of the exam, before leaving the testing center. Official score reports containing a percentile rank in each of the three major subject areas are distributed four weeks after exam completion.

General

Psychology

Psychology is the study of a human's behavior and its relation to their place on the spectrum of growth and development. An understanding of human psychology is an essential part of a certified medical assistant's (CMA's) practice because they must provide competent care to each individual patient.

Understanding Human Behavior

Behavior describes the actions an individual takes in their day-to-day lives toward others. Interpreting patient behavior, and what it means for their care, is a judgment skill a CMA must possess.

<u>Behavioral Theories</u>
The two main theories that are often used to categorize and interpret human behavior are those of psychologists Abraham Maslow (developed in 1935) and Erik Erikson (1959).

Maslow
Maslow's hierarchy of human needs is a diagram in the shape of a pyramid. Each level of the pyramid represents a human need in order from the most basic on the bottom to the most complicated on the top. These needs are at the heart of human behavior and what motivates people. At the bottom are physiological needs such as food, water, warmth, and rest. A person must meet these basic needs before moving on to the next level, which is the need to feel secure and safe. The next set of needs are psychological in nature—first the need to belong and feel loved, followed by the need to be esteemed. Being esteemed entails feeling accomplished and respected. The final need at the top of the pyramid is that of self-actualization, in which a person feels they have achieved their full potential in life. This final step can include creative activities. The CMA must keep this hierarchy of needs in mind when managing a patient's care. Maslow's pyramid will assist in understanding what motivates a patient's actions and behavior.

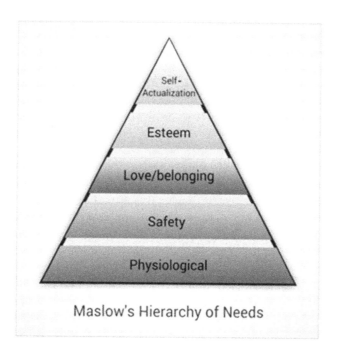

Maslow's Hierarchy of Needs

Erikson

Erikson developed eight stages a person must pass through, from birth to death, that encompass their growth and development as an individual. Each stage names a virtue that is developed if the crisis of ego is overcome successfully.

- **Birth–18 months:** In the first year and a half of a child's life, they will develop **trust vs. mistrust**, based off the nurture they receive from their parents. *Hope* is the product of proper nurture and trust. If they do not receive proper care, mistrust, along with insecurity and a feeling of worthlessness, may develop.

- **Ages 2–3:** Between the ages of two and three, the child will work through **autonomy vs. shame**. The parents must guide the child through their attempts at being independent so that *autonomy* can develop. When this happens, the child develops will. Without proper guidance, whether too permissive or too strict, the child cannot find a sense of autonomy, and shame develops.

- **Ages 4–5:** A child aged four to five will go through the **initiative vs. guilt** stage of development. This involves a modeling behavior of adults. Parents must be supportive of this initiative stage to help the child develop *purpose*. Without this encouragement of initiative, the child will feel guilt, leading to inhibition.

- **Ages 6–12:** Ages six to twelve are defined by **industry vs. inferiority**. Industry involves the capability to learn, create, and build skills and knowledge. Imagination and impulsive behavior must be tamed to develop *competence*. If the child does not move through this stage properly, inferiority develops.

- **Ages 13–19:** The thirteen- to nineteen-year-old must grapple with the crisis of **identity vs. role confusion**. A teen may experiment with different identities, most likely going through identity crises. If the crises are navigated successfully, the person develops *fidelity*, an ability to have relationships with many different people of different value systems. Failure to resolve an identity crisis results in identity diffusion and role confusion, or failure to "fit in" in a satisfactory way with the society around them. This sometimes may manifest itself in fanaticism.

- **Ages 20–24:** From age twenty to twenty-four, the young adult will work though the crisis of **intimacy vs. isolation**, in which they can have close relationships and develop *love*. Failure to do so results in isolation, in which a person is either promiscuous or exclusive. With promiscuity, the person becomes too intimate, too quickly, with many different people, but no loving relationships develop. The opposite may occur, termed *exclusivity,* in which the person rejects all relationships and those in them.

- **Ages 25–64:** This is the stage in which a person goes through the crisis of **generativity vs. stagnation**. With generativity, the person feels satisfied with the work they have completed in their lifetime. They may feel successful, having developed a legacy of which they can be proud. This develops the virtue of *caring*, manifested by caring for future generations and free giving. If this generativity has not occurred, the person will feel stagnant. This stagnation is marked by little contribution to society, meaninglessness, and potentially a midlife crisis.

- **Age 65–death:** From age sixty-five to death, the developmental stage is **integrity vs. despair**. Integrity involves an acceptance of one's accomplishments and the development of *wisdom*. If integrity does not develop, despair results, entailing a dread of death. If the person develops too much wisdom, they may display presumption. On the opposite hand, too little wisdom results in disdain, or contempt toward others and life.

<u>Defense Mechanisms</u>
Defense mechanisms in human beings can refer to either a physical response, such as the immune system's response to infections, or a mental response involving a behavioral pattern when one's emotional balance is threatened. The latter will be the defense mechanisms discussed here.

Common Types
There are many well-known, well-studied defense mechanisms, ranging from primitive to mature, that human beings exhibit. Primitive reactions can be effective in the moment but damaging in the long run, while more mature reactions are healthier and better for relationships.

- **Denial:** One of the common primitive defense mechanisms, denial is when a person rejects a reality to protect themselves from having to process it emotionally. For example, a patient may have received a diagnosis of a terminal, untreatable cancer but refuse to acknowledge the reality of their condition to avoid the painful emotions that might accompany it.

- **Undoing:** A less primitive defense mechanism, undoing involves a person trying to right a wrong they have done to someone they care about. For example, after saying something hurtful to a child, a father might heap praise upon the child and take him out to get ice cream to undo the pain of the earlier statement.

- **Sublimation:** Sublimation is an example of a mature defense mechanism. A person is sublimating when they redirect the energy they once might have put into a negative activity or impulse into something more positive and productive. Someone who might have the impulse to cheat on their significant other but does not actually want to may instead focus that energy into exercise and meditation.

Recognition and Management
It is part of the CMA's responsibility to be aware of these psychological aspects of the patient's care. Knowledge of Maslow's hierarchy of needs is important in categorizing human needs. Erikson's stages of psychological development are helpful in pointing out what ego conflict a person is going through as well as what virtues have developed. Being able to recognize common defense mechanisms and how to work through them is vital, especially in heavily emotional situations that may arise during a patient's care.

Human Growth and Development

Along with psychological development, there are specific physical stages of growth and development that each patient must go through. Depending on where the CMA practices, whether with a pediatric, geriatric, or general population, knowing these patterns and milestones will help guide decisions regarding the patient's care.

Normal Developmental Patterns/Milestones

In the first year of life, the human baby goes from being completely helpless to being able to walk, talk, and feed themselves. Here is a short list of important milestones to watch out for in the first year, as well as milestones for up to five years of age:

- **2 months:** Begins to smile, uses hand sucking to self-soothe, looks at parents, makes cooing noises, notes faces, becomes fussy when bored, and holds head up while on tummy.

- **4 months:** Spontaneously smiles and laughs, babbles, reaches for toys, and pushes legs down when held in standing position on a hard surface.

- **6 months:** Recognizes familiar faces, makes consonant sounds, puts objects in mouth, and rolls over both ways.

- **9 months:** Exhibits fear of strangers, understands the word "no," plays peek-a-boo, and gets into sitting position and sits without support.

- **1 year:** Displays nervousness around strangers and cries when parents leave, waves "hi" or "bye," puts things in and out of a container, and may take steps or even walk.

- **18 months:** Has temper tantrums, points to objects they want, says single words, understands functions of basic objects such as a phone, and carries toys while walking.

- **2 years:** Copies the behavior of others, knows names of familiar body parts such as "nose," begins sorting colors and shapes, and kicks a ball.

- **3 years:** Shows concern for crying friend, follows two- or three-step instructions, does three- to four-piece puzzles, runs easily, and climbs.

- **4 years:** Enjoys group play and storytelling, names colors and numbers, and stands on one foot for up to 2 seconds.

- **5 years:** Mimics friends; enjoys singing, dancing, and acting; speaks more clearly; counts to ten or higher; and stands on one foot for 10 seconds or longer.

Death and Dying Stages

Stages of Grief

In 1969, Swiss psychiatrist Elisabeth Kubler-Ross developed the five stages of grief, in which mourners ultimately accept the reality of their imminent death. This can also apply to family members dealing with a loss. The Kubler-Ross stages begin with denial, followed by anger, bargaining, depression, and finally acceptance.

- Denial: In this stage, the person denies the reality of their or their loved one's terminal prognosis, refusing to accept it.

- Anger: After reality has set in, the person is filled with anger at the situation, feeling helpless.

- Bargaining: This stage entails a sort of negotiation between the grieving and a higher power, looking to trade one thing for the restoral of their loved one to health.

- Depression: After bargaining has failed, the person becomes depressed, feeling hopeless, lacking motivation, and lacking interest in any sort of positive, healing activities.

- Acceptance: The final stage, which not everyone reaches, is accepting the loss of the loved one and moving on with a positive perspective.

These stages have been debated and are somewhat controversial, as it is not an exact roadmap of each patient's emotional experience. They are, however, a helpful guide the CMA can use as a reference point when assessing a patient's emotional response to their or a loved one's mortality in the case of a terminal diagnosis.

Signs of active death: There are several signs a CMA should look for to determine if a patient is dying. A patient may spend most of their time sleeping, spending less and less time awake. The patient may become confused, disoriented, and even experience hallucinations, indicating the neurological system is no longer functioning properly. They may become withdrawn socially. Physical signs include labored breathing, including the "death rattle," in which a patient is unable to clear secretions in the airway, the telltale sign that death is near. Decreased appetite, bowel movements, and urination are the result of the gastrointestinal (GI) system ceasing activity. Mottling and coolness in the extremities are evidence that circulation is slowing as the body shuts itself down. The role of the CMA, depending on their practice setting, is to support the patient and family during this difficult time. Making the patient comfortable using whatever resources are available is the best intervention to ensure a peaceful passing.

Communication

The CMA must develop strong communication skills adapted to a variety of different types of patients to expedite and facilitate the best possible care. The following are various types of communication and populations with which a CMA will interact in their practice.

Therapeutic/Adaptive Responses to Diverse Populations

Visually Impaired
A patient with a visual impairment will require adaptations to the CMA's communications techniques to ensure a clear message is sent and received. The CMA should identify themselves clearly when beginning their assessment. The CMA should never treat the patient who has a visual impairment as if they have a deficit in intellect or as if they are deaf. The CMA should check the environment to make sure there are no distractions, such as a loud TV, that may make it difficult to be heard. The CMA should ask questions to ensure the message has been received and understood by the patient. Assessing the level of visual impairment will assist in knowing how much assistance the patient will need. Someone who is legally blind versus someone with complete vision loss from birth will have different needs for assistance.

Deaf and Hard of Hearing
When communicating with persons who are deaf or hard of hearing, an important first step is to assess the level of hearing loss. This will guide further communication. Depending on the amount of hearing loss, lip reading, visual tools, hearing aids, an increased volume of the CMA's voice, or the hiring of a sign language interpreter may or may not be useful. The CMA should directly face the person with a hearing impairment when addressing them so that understanding can be better assessed. The CMA should not be in another room, have their back to the patient, or compete with a loud TV or other distraction while

trying to communicate. The CMA may ask the patient questions to ensure understanding of the message.

<u>Age-Specific</u>
There are considerations to be made regarding the age of the person the CMA is communicating with.

Geriatric
Geriatric refers to an older adult, a population of patients the CMA may work with quite frequently. The CMA should remember that active listening is as important as, if not more important than, speaking as far as communication goes. The CMA should ask questions but listen intently to the answers to ascertain if the patient understands. The CMA needs to remember that interrupting is rude and can compromise trust and good communication. The CMA should take their time when giving instructions, ensuring understanding. It is not wise to use jargon, slang, or other language that the geriatric patient may not understand. If the patient needs to use new technology such as an online patient account, an assessment of Internet usage and proficiency would be useful.

Pediatric
There are a few tricks a CMA should have up their sleeve when addressing a pediatric patient to make them feel comfortable and safe in a medical environment. The CMA should address the child by name to create a tone of familiarity. Getting down to the child's level physically—in other words, squatting down to eye level—will help the child feel they are on the same level as their caregiver, rather than the CMA towering over them. Smiling and exuding a positive attitude will create the right environment for the CMA to care for the child. Making medical tools and equipment into toys when appropriate, such as gloves or tongue depressors, can help the child feel at ease. The CMA should enlist the parents as team members in the child's care.

Adolescent
Communicating with teenagers can present its own unique challenges for the CMA. No longer a child and not quite an adult, the adolescent must feel they are part of the care team and that they have a say in decision making. It may be useful to conduct interviews with adolescents without their parents being present, if possible. This will help when trying to conduct a frank discussion on the patient's sexual activity as well as potential drug/alcohol usage. The assessment of an adolescent should include questions about mental health issues, such as depression and anxiety. The teen may feel more comfortable discussing these issues without their parent present, though the parent should be made a member of the team when addressing any issues that are discovered. Another important topic to approach with teens is stress, its causes, and coping mechanisms. In some cases, it is important to inform the adolescent which topics will remain confidential. This may encourage them to share more with the CMA.

<u>Seriously/Terminally Ill</u>
Navigating the tricky area of communicating with a patient who is diagnosed with a terminal illness can present a real challenge to the CMA. It is important to be honest with the patient. The CMA should be an active listener, looking for opportunities to connect the patient with valuable resources and support. The CMA should offer compassion but not false hope. The CMA may want to say something meaningful or helpful, but this is not always the best option. Sometimes simply being present, offering a hug, or holding a patient's hand is better than any words. The CMA should also look for opportunities to communicate with and support the family of the terminally ill patient. After the patient passes, they will need guidance to bereavement, loss, and grief resources.

Intellectual Disability

A patient with an intellectual disability may need additional help communicating with the health care team. The CMA will need to practice patience and allow extra time for communicating messages with and receiving messages from a person with an intellectual disability. The CMA should work with caregivers to get helpful tips for working with a patient. Every patient is different, and a full-time caregiver or loved one will know what works best when trying to communicate with the patient. The CMA should try to explain care in the simplest terms possible, avoiding complicated medical jargon. The CMA should focus on the patient's strengths rather than pointing out and focusing on weaknesses. As with all communication, the CMA should concentrate on being an active listener, open to receiving the patient's concerns and giving them time to voice them.

Illiterate

A person who is illiterate cannot read and/or write. It is not always apparent to a CMA which patients may have this problem. There is a type of illiteracy called *health illiteracy* in which a patient is highly unfamiliar with medical information and is, therefore, unable to apply it to their own health and health care management. In illiteracy and health illiteracy, asking questions and listening for comprehension are both tools the CMA can use to determine how well the patient understands their individual health care plan. If a patient cannot read or write, the CMA can offer their health information to them in a different format. The CMA can read through instructions for home care and ensure that a literate caregiver is accessible to the patient to assist them with written materials. Patients with low health care literacy tend to make their health care decisions based on emotions and practical considerations such as if they will be able to get a ride to the doctor. An example of emotional decision making would be a patient who doesn't go to the doctor because he "doesn't like needles"; this is irrational, since not every doctor visit implies needles, yet it creates a barrier to successful health care. Identifying these barriers is the first step to overcoming illiteracy.

Non-English Speaking

In the case of a non-English-speaking patient, the CMA should seek out translation services. This can come from a family member who accompanies the patient or possibly be provided by the facility where the CMA works. Seeking educational materials in the patient's native tongue will be helpful in clearly communicating with the patient after they leave the facility.

Anxious/Angry/Distraught

If a patient appears to be having an emotional response to care, such as anxiety or anger, the CMA may act to assist the patient to a calmer state. Determining the cause of the emotional reaction is the first step. This can be determined through question asking and active listening. The next step would be to eliminate any stimulus that might be upsetting the patient. Taking note of the response in the medical record to avoid future confrontations will assist future caregivers.

Socially/Culturally/Ethnically Diverse

The CMA must be competent in culturally sensitive care toward people of many different backgrounds. The CMA must first check their own feelings and biases about people who are different from themselves to treat these people fairly. Everyone has the right to fair and quality health care. The best thing a CMA can do when presented with someone of a different background is to offer respect, give dignified care, and ask questions before proceeding to avoid any unnecessary offense.

Nonverbal Communication

The CMA not only communicates with their words but also with their body language. Knowing what one is communicating nonverbally and taking care to send the right message is vital to quality patient care.

<u>Body Language</u>
- **Posture:** Slouching indicates disinterest, fatigue, and disengagement. The CMA should have erect posture, not only for the health benefit, but to show the patient they are engaged in their care.

- **Position:** The CMA should be facing the patient, both their face and body. Not facing the patient indicates the CMA does not care about sending a good message and that they do not care about their situation.

- **Facial expression:** It is not necessary for the CMA to have a big, bright smile on their face at all times, but a pleasant expression that is responsive to the patient's own facial expression gives off a positive energy that the patient may find encouraging.

- **Territoriality/physical boundaries:** Different cultures have different boundaries that are considered acceptable. The CMA should maintain a respectful distance from the patient, never too far away or too close for comfort. The patient's reaction is a good measure of whether the CMA is at an appropriate distance.

- **Gestures:** Most people use hand gestures to help communicate a message. The CMA may use hand gestures but must be aware of how much they are doing this. The CMA should avoid overgesturing, as this will take away from their overall message.

- **Touch:** Therapeutic touch is appropriate in certain instances with certain patients. This could involve touching their hand, putting one hand on their shoulder, or even a hug. Caution should be used when employing therapeutic touch, as some patients might find this uncomfortable. The CMA should use their best judgment on when this type of intervention is most appropriate and helpful.

- **Mannerisms:** Everyone has certain unique mannerisms, or a way they speak or gesture. The CMA should be aware of their own quirks and idiosyncrasies if possible and make certain they do not interfere with the patient's care or cause offense.

- **Eye contact:** Good eye contact is crucial to good patient care. Not enough eye contact shows lack of interest and boredom; too much eye contact can be construed as weird and scary. The CMA should be aware of their eye contact and use it as a listening tool to properly tune in to the patient's message they are trying to send.

Communication Cycle

An understanding of the basics of communication, involving the communication cycle, is important for the CMA to know to communicate effectively with their patients.

Sender-Message-Receiver Feedback
The communication cycle starts with a sender. The sender sends the message to the receiver and looks for feedback. This goes on and on through a circular cycle until transmission is ended, such as the end of a conversation.

Listening Skills
Active/Therapeutic
One of the best communication skills the CMA can employ is active or therapeutic listening. This involves being especially engaged when the patient is sending their message back to the CMA. Listening carefully allows the CMA to better sync care with the patient's unique needs. Failure to listen properly will result in conflicts with the patient's care.

Assess Level of Understanding
The CMA must be able to assess the patient's level of understanding. This can be ascertained by the following four techniques:

- **Reflection:** Reflection is to paraphrase what a patient says, allowing both the patient and the CMA to come to an agreement about what was said.

- **Restatement:** Restatement is repeating what a patient has just said back to them.

- **Clarification:** Clarification is to make clear; in this instance, it means to offer back the essential message the patient has given along with any questions the CMA may have.

- **Feedback:** After clarifying the patient's meaning, the CMA may give feedback, or a reaction to their message that improves the relationship and further communications.

Barriers to Communication
The CMA may run into barriers to communication, whether internal or external, that will degrade the quality of communication or even break down communication entirely. Identifying these barriers is the first step to overcoming them to restore effective communication.

Internal Distractions
- **Pain:** If a patient is in pain, their ability to communicate will break down. Treating the pain first will facilitate communication between the patient and the health care team.

- **Hunger:** A patient who is hungry will have difficulty concentrating on sending and receiving messages effectively. In some instances, it is impossible to avoid a hungry patient, as many must fast for tests and procedures. Alleviating hunger, where possible, will ensure better communication.

- **Anger:** If there is something angering a patient, this could pose a potential blockade to effective communication. Identifying the inflammatory stimulus and working toward a resolution will improve future communications with the patient.

External/Environmental Distractions

- **Temperature:** A patient who is distracted by feeling too hot or too cold will have difficulty maintaining a normal conversation with the CMA. Warm blankets for a cold patient and fans/open windows/air conditioning for a hot patient are helpful for fixing this problem.

- **Noise:** The CMA would be wise to eliminate unnecessary noise when communicating with a patient. This may entail closing the door of the patient's room to block hallway chatter and/or turning a TV's volume down.

Collection of Data

The CMA must be able to ask questions that collect information from the patient necessary for their care.

Types of Questions
Exploratory
An exploratory question seeks to explore different possibilities with the patient on a specific subject. Usually a subject has been established, and the CMA is seeking to find further information about the subject. It is a type of open-ended question.

Open-Ended
An open-ended question is one in which the receiver cannot simply answer "yes" or "no." They must explain themselves, thus making it a more revealing way to communicate. This is good for beginning a conversation.

Closed/Direct
A closed question can be answered simply with a "yes" or a "no." This type of question is good for gathering a lot of simple data quickly.

Telephone Techniques

At times, the CMA may be called upon to handle phone calls in a practice setting, using triage techniques as well as providing information to the callers.

Call Management
Screening/Gathering Data
The CMA must be able to collect data from the caller to screen them and direct them to the proper outlet. This ensures an office is run smoothly.

Emergency/Urgent Situations
The CMA must be aware of how to handle emergency calls and urgent situations. These situations may be handled on the phone, or it may be necessary to redirect the caller to emergency services for situation resolution.

Messages
Taking Messages
When taking a message, the CMA must be able to gather the appropriate information about the caller, why they called, and who needs to receive their information. Too much or too little data will result in mishandled situations and conflicts that will require more work to resolve in the future.

Leaving Messages

The CMA will need to leave messages at times for both patients and health care providers. Providing succinct information in the message is appropriate. Again, too much or too little information will result in further conflicts to be handled in the future.

Interpersonal Skills

Displaying Impartial Conduct

Along with providing culturally competent care, the CMA must be able to treat people of all different backgrounds and lifestyle choices. Awareness of one's own biases and prejudices is the first step, followed by a conscious effort to provide dignified and respectful care to all.

Recognizing Stereotypes and Biases

Self-awareness is an important tool that a CMA must employ to assess their own feelings about people who are different from themselves. Armed with this self-knowledge, the CMA may then be more aware of any partialities they may be displaying toward people of the same background vs. impartiality toward people who are different from them. All patients coming to the CMA seeking quality health care have a right to impartial treatment, without bias, judgment, or prejudice.

Demonstrating Empathy/Sympathy/Compassion

An important virtue that all members of the health care team, including the CMA, must exhibit is compassion. This involves an empathetic or sympathetic response to pain and suffering and a desire to seek resolution through medical interventions and support. Without this basic reaction of compassion, health care is void of any real meaning or reward for either party involved. The CMA must seek the good of their patients, through healthy communication and effective problem solving.

Professionalism

In the profession of medical assisting, a certain code of conduct, competence, and skill is expected. The CMA must exhibit the following professional behavior to be an esteemed member of the profession.

Professional Behavior

Professional Situations

Every situation involving an interaction with a patient or co-member of the health care team requires professional behavior from the CMA.

Displaying Tact, Diplomacy, Courtesy, Respect, Dignity

A CMA shows professionalism by showing tact, or sensitivity and skill, when interacting with others. A diplomatic approach involves this same sensitivity to preserve and grow a relationship. Every person should be shown respect and dignity as part of a professional's behavior.

Demonstrating Responsibility, Integrity/Honesty

A CMA who is perceived as honest and responsible will win the trust of their patients and peers. Distrust is a direct result of dishonest behavior and a lack of integrity.

Responding to Criticism

A CMA will show their true professional colors when they respond to criticism. The professional response is to see criticism as a challenge and an opportunity to grow, rather than an attack and unfair blow. When a member of a profession responds appropriately to criticism with humility and an open mind, they are afforded the opportunity to better themselves in their profession.

Professional Image
It has been said that an individual should dress for the job they wish to do. This applies to the CMA in that they should be careful to present the right image of themselves to others. The CMA is a representative of a respected medical profession, and conduct should be performed as such. The CMA should dress themselves, groom themselves, and present themselves, in public and on social media, in a way that is consistent with their profession. Failure to do so may result in lost respect from peers and patients as well as a tarnishing of the title of CMA.

Performing as a Team Member

The CMA is a part of the health care team. This team includes doctors, nurses, and other specialists. Being able to cooperate and collaborate with the CMA's fellow team members is part of excellent patient care.

Principles of Health Care Team Dynamics
Cooperation for Optimal Outcomes
The goal of health care is to take care of the patient. When the patient is the center of care and this goal is the highest priority, high-quality health care will be delivered. This requires cooperation and respect between the different specialists working with the patient. Clear communication is essential in delivering high-quality care to the patient. When one member of the team fails to listen to another team member's contributions and thoughts regarding the patient's care, an important consideration could be missed to the detriment of the patient's care. It is also important that the CMA respects the authority of those team members with a higher level of education and training.

Identification of the Roles and Credentials of Health Care Team Members
The CMA will work with several different specialists, most commonly nurses, doctors, and certified nurses' aides, among many others.

- **CNA:** A certified nurse assistant (CNA) is a member of the team who reports directly to a nurse. They must complete four to twelve weeks of classroom and clinical training along with passing a state certification test. Their role is to perform many of the caregiving activities with the patient, such as bathing, feeding, and taking vital signs, though some roles of a CNA will overlap with that of a CMA depending on the place of practice and facility policy.

- **RN:** A registered nurse (RN) is a member of the team in charge of the patient's care plan as well as taking and carrying out physician orders. RNs have either a two-year or four-year degree along with passing national boards.

- **MD:** The CMA will report directly to a doctor in charge of the patient's care. MDs in the United States generally have four years of undergraduate, four years of medical school, and between three and seven years of residency to achieve licensure in the practice of medicine. MDs will diagnose and prescribe a treatment plan for the patient.

Time Management Principles
The CMA will have many demands on their time. It is vital that they practice good time management to provide the highest quality of care to patients.

Prioritizing Responsibilities

To manage time effectively, the CMA must first be able to prioritize tasks. For example, the most important tasks must be recognized as such and completed in a timely manner. Being aware of how long a task takes will assist in scheduling a CMA's day and planning how to proceed.

Medical Law/Regulatory Guidelines

The CMA should be aware of the following medical law and regulatory guidelines and how they apply to their daily practice.

Advance Directives

An advance directive is a legal document that a patient draws up to ensure their wishes are honored even if they are unable to make their own decisions due to an incapacitating health care condition.

Living Will

A living will is a legal document that allows a patient to make clear their wishes regarding different medical decisions should they become incapacitated in some way and unable to make these decisions. Part of a living will can name a person to make medical decisions for the patient, though a living will is not the same as a medical durable power of attorney.

Medical Durable Power of Attorney

A power of attorney document names a patient-appointed representative to make health care decisions on their behalf should they become incapacitated. The difference between this document and the living will is that the living will is more focused on end-of-life care, while the power of attorney can span a longer period and can end when the patient regains the ability to make their own decisions.

Patient Self-Determination Act (PSDA)

This act, passed in 1990, mandates that health care facilities inform and protect a patient's right to make decisions about their care. This right extends even if they become incapacitated through advance directives such as the living will and power of attorney.

Uniform Anatomical Gift Act (UAGA)

Passed originally in 1968, then again with revisions in 1987 and 2006, the UAGA is a legal framework for the donation and use of organs, tissues, and other human anatomy in the United States. These "anatomical gifts" are used in medical practice, for scientific research, and for educational purposes.

Occupational Safety and Health Administration (OSHA)

OSHA is an agency that was developed under the Occupational Safety and Health Act in 1970 under President Nixon's administration. OSHA works to ensure the health and safety of American workers through regulations, laws, and their enforcement.

Food and Drug Administration (FDA)

In 1906, the FDA was formed to regulate food safety in the United States. This involves supervising and controlling products such as tobacco, dietary supplements, medications, vaccines, and many other products that are consumed by the American population. The FDA's oversight extends even to products consumed by animals such as their feed and veterinary products.

Clinical Laboratory Improvement Act (CLIA 1988)

CLIA is a series of federal standards set in place to regulate the testing of human specimens in laboratories. These specimens, which can include blood, tissue, and other bodily material, can be used to diagnose, prevent, and treat various diseases. Regulation is necessary to ensure high standards of quality are followed in clinical laboratories.

Americans With Disabilities Act Amendments Act (ADAAA)

Passed in 2008, the ADAAA amends a previous act, the ADA, to better define what "disability" means for certain Americans as well as protecting and upholding the rights of those with disabilities in the United States. The ADAAA was a response to several Supreme Court decisions that were thought to have limited the rights of those with disabilities.

Health Insurance Portability and Accountability Act (HIPAA)

Signed into law in 1996 by President Bill Clinton, this law protects patient privacy and improves access to care.

Health Insurance Portability Access and Renewal Without Preexisting Conditions
This part of HIPAA allows employees to switch jobs and keep health insurance despite preexisting conditions. HIPAA aimed to decrease paperwork and reduce inefficiencies within the health insurance industry.

Coordination of Care to Prevent Duplication of Services
By reducing the amount of human effort and paperwork used to process claims, HIPAA sought to streamline the entire process to prevent errors, duplications, and fraud.

Health Information Technology for Economic and Clinical Health (HITECH) Act

HITECH was signed into law in 2009 under the Obama administration. Under this act, health care providers would be incentivized to adopt new technology that put health care records into an electronic database, thus streamlining patient case management.

Patient's Right to Inspect, Amend, and Restrict Access to Their Medical Record
Under this act, a patient has the right to access and maintain the confidentiality of their health care records.

Drug Enforcement Agency (DEA)

The DEA was created under the Nixon administration in 1973 as part of a "war on drugs." The DEA's mission is to combat drug abuse and drug trafficking through investigation, apprehension, and prosecution programs.

Controlled Substances Act of 1970
In 1970, President Nixon signed this act to regulate the use and distribution of certain drugs. This act includes a list of "schedules," I–V, that categorizes each type of drug and their potential for abuse. For example, Schedule I drugs, such as heroin, are considered a high risk for abuse.

Medical Assistant Scope of Practice

The CMA needs to be aware of what they are and are not allowed to do, referred to as their *scope of practice.* A CMA must respect patient privacy and confidentiality. A CMA must practice culturally competent care, display professionalism in all situations, adhere to risk management and safety policies, and perform office management duties such as maintaining patient records, taking and receiving phone calls, and other official health care communications. The CMA is responsible for documenting information about the patient in their health care record, including observations, clinical treatments, and vital signs. Each state has different guidelines on the exact duties and responsibilities of CMAs, but every CMA is responsible for knowing what is legally within their scope of practice.

Consequences of Failing to Operate Within Scope
Operating outside of a CMA's scope of practice can result in disciplinary action or even loss of licensure.

Genetic Information Nondiscrimination Act (GINA) of 2008

In 2008, Congress enacted GINA to prevent employers and health insurers from discriminating against people based on their genetic information. Genetic discrimination means to discriminate against a person based on defects or perceived defects in their DNA.

Centers for Disease Control and Prevention (CDC)

The CDC is a federal agency that promotes public health through disease control and prevention initiatives. Their mission is protecting the health security of the nation.

Consumer Protection Acts

These acts are regulations that promote free trade, protect the consumer from misinformation and fraud, and promote competition.

Fair Debt Collection Practices Act
This act protects consumers from being harassed by debt collectors. Debt collectors may not use abusive, unfair, or deceiving techniques when attempting to collect from debtors.

Truth in Lending Act (TILA) of 1968 (Regulation Z)
TILA's primary purpose was to inform consumers before they sign up for a line of credit. Creditors must inform the consumer of the terms and conditions.

Public Health and Welfare Disclosure

Entities in the United States that provide health care are required to disclose certain information to public health authorities, such as state health departments, the CDC, and the FDA. This disclosure of information, which is usually the least possible required, is used for the interest of public health and fighting the spread of disease.

Public Health Statutes
Public health authorities are mandated to fight illness and its spread and reduce the number of deaths in the nation.

Communicable Diseases
Entities must disclose information about communicable diseases to public health authorities to prevent the spread of disease in a community or nation. The information is usually reduced to the minimum of what is needed to protect the privacy of patients.

Vital Statistics
Birth records, birth rates, and death records are examples of vital statistics that must be disclosed to public health authorities for tracking and monitoring the population.

Abuse/Neglect/Exploitation Against Child/Elder
Entities that discover abuse or neglect in a child or elderly person must report this mandatorily in the interest of the abused. This may be done without the authorization of the victim.

If domestic abuse is likewise suspected, it also must be reported to the proper authorities. In some cases, this is the local police department. The police department is authorized to receive and respond to such reports.

Wounds of Violence
Domestic, child, and elder abuse leave damaging and long-lasting psychological wounds on their victims that remain long after any physical wounds have healed. These internal wounds have an effect not only on the victim but also children and other relationships in the victim's life. Recognizing that abuse may be occurring and reporting it appropriately is part of the CMA's role as a patient advocate. These wounds cannot heal until the problem is acknowledged.

Confidentiality

One basic right of a patient is confidentiality. Confidentiality means that the patient's health care information will remain private. Only those involved in the patient's direct care will have access to their records for the use of diagnosing and treating illness. A breach of confidentiality is a serious offense that could lead to disciplinary action.

Electronic Access Audit/Activity Log
Most of the patient's health information will be logged in an electronic health record. Anyone who accesses this information will be tracked and monitored. Routinely, most institutions will conduct audits to see who has been accessing which records and if they were authorized to do so.

Use and Disclosure of Personal/Protected Health Information (PHI)
Consent/Authorization to Release
A patient is usually asked to sign a consent to release PHI before receiving treatment. This allows the health care provider to release their information for treatment, payment, and health care operations, abbreviated to TPO. Treatment is all care given to the patient by the health care provider; payment involves claims, billing, and collection by insurance companies; and health care operations involves educational purposes such as training new CMAs. Health care operations does not include using patient information for research; a different consent must be signed for that purpose.

Drug and Alcohol Treatment Records
Certain patient health records regarding the treatment of drug and alcohol addictions are specifically protected by federal regulations. Violation of the confidentiality of these records could result in a criminal penalty to the offender. There are certain emergency situations in which this information may be shared as well as research purposes in which release of information is allowed.

HIV-Related Information

HIV-related information is protected by law. Reports on diagnoses and treatments are to be kept private and confidential by health care providers. The reason this information is kept confidential is that persons with an HIV-AIDS diagnosis may face discrimination because of some people's unfair prejudices.

Mental Health Records

Part of HIPAA provides special protection to mental health records. For example, though mental health information is largely grouped together with general health information about a patient, psychotherapy notes have special safeguards that keep them confidential. In the case of minors with mental health issues, there are specific guidelines that dictate who can be talked to about which issues, such as discussing a teen's medication regimen for mental illness with a legal guardian or parent.

Health Care Rights and Responsibilities

There are several different lists that have been drawn up to define a patient's health care rights. Some are legal and others informal. Each one, whether the hospice patient's bill of rights or an individual state's lists of rights, has key features in common. These key features are usually a right to informed consent, respect, nondiscrimination, and confidentiality of patient information, among other things. Each person also has the responsibility to take care of their own health as well as respecting health care workers. The idea of a patient bill of rights is to empower the patient, encouraging them to take an active role in their relationship with health care providers. Every citizen of the United States has certain health care rights defended by federal law. The most recent modification to health care rights in the United States was the Affordable Care Act (ACA) of 2010, signed into law by President Barack Obama.

Patient's Bill of Rights/Patient Care Partnership

Typically, a patient's bill of rights will include the following: easy access to one's own medical records, a choice of providers and insurance plans, accessibility to care, an active role in the health care team, a right to be respected, a right to dignified and nondiscriminatory care, and confidentiality of patient health information. The patient is a partner in the health care team and should be treated as such.

Professional Liability

To be liable means to be responsible for something in a legal sense. As a member of the CMA profession, a CMA has legal obligations called *professional liability* that may arise if they commit a serious error. Usually this takes the form of money owed to a patient filing a lawsuit for some sort of negligent act on the part of the professional. Legal penalties could be as severe as losing one's license to practice.

Current Standard of Care

The CMA must stay within their scope of practice and always meet current care standards to avoid the consequences of malpractice. Each state has specific guidelines defining a CMA's scope of practice. In most states, a CMA may administer medications, perform office administrative duties, assist an MD with office procedures, draw blood, and prepare a patient for examination, among other assistive-type duties. A CMA generally cannot independently triage, diagnose, or treat a patient. If a CMA makes an error involving independent diagnosis and treatment of a patient that results in patient harm, the CMA will most certainly be liable and subject to legal penalties.

Standards of Conduct

A CMA is expected to conduct themselves professionally, under the guidance and direct supervision of an MD. Failure to meet proper conduct standards will result in disciplinary action and perhaps loss of licensure, as well as being a poor reflection of what the profession of medical assisting aspires to be.

Malpractice Coverage

There is insurance coverage to help offset the costs of potential liabilities called *malpractice insuranc*e. This insurance may be purchased by individuals through the insurer of their choice. Malpractice insurance may also be available through one's place of employment as part of a group plan. It is up to the individual CMA to determine if they should purchase malpractice insurance, as litigation can be quite costly if handled alone.

Consent to Treat

Informed Consent

An important part of the patient's bill of rights is informed consent. This means the patient has been adequately informed about their health care plan, whether that involves new medications, vaccinations, procedures, diagnostic screenings, and so on. The patient is granting their permission to go ahead with the care plan after being properly educated about it. It is up to the health care team to obtain this informed consent. This usually takes the form of a patient-signed document that goes in the permanent health care record.

Implied Consent

This type of consent does not involve the patient signing a document or even verbally granting permission, but rather it is assumed that any reasonable person would consent to the health care interventions being performed. The most common use of implied consent is in emergency situations, in which lifesaving interventions are necessary and there is not enough time to perform informed consent with the patient, such as cardiopulmonary resuscitation (CPR) after cardiac arrest.

Expressed Consent

This type of consent entails that the patient consent to a medical intervention either verbally, nonverbally through a gesture such as a nod, or in writing. This type of consent differs from informed consent in that there is not necessarily an education process that precedes it. This type of consent generally requires a witness.

Patient Incompetence

A patient who is unable to make their own informed decisions about their health care plan is termed *incompetent*. In the case of an incompetent patient, it may be necessary to use a proxy, such as a power of attorney, to make health care decisions for them.

Emancipated Minor

If a minor is legally emancipated, it means they are freed from having parental consent to certain things. The legal age for emancipation is generally sixteen. A patient may be medically emancipated if they become pregnant, thus freeing them to give consent with associated medical procedures and maintaining confidentiality of their records at that point.

Mature Minor

The mature minor concept applies to unemancipated minors and says that if a patient is deemed mature enough and the medical intervention is not especially serious, they may make their own decisions and give their own consent without parental consent.

Medicolegal Terms and Doctrines

The following is a list of common legal terms the CMA should be acquainted with should they come up in their practice.

- **Subpoena duces tecum:** This Latin term translates to "under penalty you shall bring with you." This is a legal document ordering a person to come to court and bring any relevant documents to the case.

- **Subpoena:** This simply entails the person must produce evidence for a case.

- **Respondeat superior:** This Latin term literally means "let the master answer." This legal term refers to an employer being responsible for the actions of their employees, usually used in the case of tort.

- **Res ipsa loquitur:** In Latin, this term means "the thing speaks for itself." It applies to medical malpractice where negligence is implied when an accident occurs.

- **Locum tenens:** This phrase is Latin for "one holding a place" and in medicine usually refers to one physician filling the place of another.

- **Defendant/plaintiff:** A defendant is the person against whom the plaintiff is filing a complaint or suit. A patient would be the plaintiff, and the physician would be the defendant if the patient filed a lawsuit against the physician.

- **Deposition:** A deposition is a legal statement that is recorded outside of the court, usually an oral testimony that is written down as evidence.

- **Arbitration/mediation:** Both these terms refer to a way of settling legal disputes outside of court. Arbitration is a cheaper, faster alternative to settling disputes. An arbitrator, a third party, is selected to help resolve the dispute. They decide who to award, if anyone. If one decides to go the arbitrary route, the case may not be tried in court, since it is considered legally resolved. Mediation differs from arbitration in that it is more flexible, can occur before arbitration, is more informal, and the mediator simply facilitates communication between opposing parties in search of a resolution.

- **Good Samaritan laws:** These laws protect persons who choose to assist someone in need of emergency medical assistance outside of a health care facility. If an unintended consequence results, or the person's life is not saved, the person is protected if they had good intention and offered reasonable assistance.

Categories of Law

There are four different areas of law in the United States the CMA should become acquainted with.

Criminal Law
This branch of the legal system involves consequences for those who commit crimes.

Infraction/Misdemeanor/Felony
There are varying degrees of crimes, from infractions to felonies. Infractions invoke tickets and fines. A misdemeanor can be punishable by law with up to one year of incarceration or jail time. A felony is the most serious offense, punishable with over a year in jail time.

<u>Civil Law</u>
This type of law involves the relationships between community members.

Contracts (Physician–Patient Relationships)

- **Legal obligations to the patient:** Due to the sensitive nature of information exchanged between a doctor and their patient, confidentiality is an obligation that must be honored, or there will be legal consequences.

- **Consequences for patient noncompliance:** There are some cases in which a patient becomes noncompliant, or refuses to follow medical advice regarding their care. In some cases, the physician might feel the need to protect themselves from any potential legal consequences of the patient's noncompliance, telling the patient to seek a new provider. There may be documents that the physician can have the patient sign, indicating that they were advised one way and that they refused to follow medical direction, thus freeing the physician from any liability.

- **Termination of medical care**

  o Elements/behaviors for withdrawal of care: The patient has the right to refuse to follow medical advice; however, they cannot hold the physician liable for any consequences they suffer, such as a medical emergency or worsening of their condition. The CMA and other health care staff must respect the patient's right and always treat them with respect despite difference of opinions.

  o Patient notification and documentation: It is important when terminating care of a patient to properly notify them and thoroughly document the case for legal protection.

- **Ownership of medical records:** Each state in the United States has different rules as to who owns medical records. In some states, the hospital and/or the physician has ownership; in other states, the patient owns the information; and in some states, there is no legal specification as to who owns medical records. Under HIPAA, all patients have a right to access their own medical record and may argue this legally.

Torts
A *tort* is a legal term referring to a violation of a person's rights leading to legal action.

- **Invasion of privacy:** In medicine, very private and sensitive information is exchanged between the physician and the patient. The CMA must ensure that any care given to a patient does not invade their privacy. This is easily avoided by being clear about the plan of care and obtaining the patient's consent, whether expressed, implied, or informed. Serious invasions of privacy subject to legal action include interception of private phone calls, recording conversations without the patient's knowledge, and "peeping Tom" behavior.

- **Negligence:** This type of tort indicates that action was not taken where it should have been, and a patient was harmed as a result.

- **Intentional torts**

  o **Battery:** Originating from the term "to batter," battery means to hit someone, causing injury. It can include shooting someone with a gun.

- **Assault:** This means to threaten violence against a person but stops short of actual battery.

- **Slander:** This is spoken defamation, in which someone says something about someone else that causes harm.

- **Libel:** This is the written form of defamation, in which someone writes something that damages or hurts someone else.

Statutory Law

This type of law includes all the laws that have been written down and enacted by legislative action.

Medical Practice Acts

Any law that governs the practice of medicine, usually within a state or a country, is termed a *medical practice act*.

Common Law (Legal Precedents)

Common law is based on previously decided court cases, termed *precedents*.

Medical Ethics

As in every profession, the profession of medical assisting requires that CMAs act according to a code of ethics. Ethics are a group of moral principles that define what is the right or wrong thing to do. In the case of medical ethics, this applies to treating patients and handling their care the right way.

Ethical Standards

The CMA adheres to a code of ethics like others in the medical profession, but especially to the physician who employs them. There will always be gray areas in patient care that raise ethical questions about how to proceed with the patient's care. When there is an ethical question, the CMA must respect human dignity first and foremost, maintain confidentiality, and seek to provide the greatest service to the patients they serve. These principles are part of the creed set forth by the American Association of Medical Assistants (AAMA).

Factors Affecting Ethical Decisions

Legal

An ethical decision may have legal factors such as what actions the CMA takes that are within their legal scope of practice. An example would be a patient with a terminal illness wishing to take a euthanasia approach. Euthanasia, sometimes called "physician-assisted suicide," is a process by which a patient with a terminal illness ends their own life instead of letting the illness take its course. This can be assisted by a physician or not. It is also sometimes called "death with dignity." There are some states in the United States in which euthanasia is currently legal and others in which it is not. The CMA can always consult with their supervising physician or even with professional associations to seek answers to such dilemmas.

Moral

A situation might arise in which the CMA is morally conflicted as to how to proceed. This may involve a suspicion that a colleague is doing something illegal, such as stealing controlled substances to feed a drug addiction. The CMA may want to ignore it, since it seems this colleague is still able to carry out their duties, but on the other hand, they know that the addiction might become worse or the colleague may make a serious medical error while under the influence, causing patient harm. It is the ethical duty of the CMA to do the right thing in all circumstances, upholding the care of the patients above all else.

Risk Management, Quality Assurance, and Safety

Risk management teams work in hospitals to prevent adverse events from happening to health care workers. Health care workers such as CMAs face a variety of hazards in their workplace, from blood-borne pathogens and infectious diseases to exposure to radiation and other harmful substances. Preventing accidents and promoting the health and safety of health care workers is a high priority for risk managers to ensure that a high quality of health care is provided to the patients.

Workplace Accident Prevention

Slips/Trips/Falls

This area of risk management involves the external environment in which the CMA works. A good housekeeping team and grounds crew will ensure most of these types of accidents do not happen. Slips/trips/falls can result in injuries that take the employee out of the workforce for a time or indefinitely. Falls can occur anywhere in a health care facility, including hallways, doorways, ramps, heavy traffic areas, stairs, unstable work surfaces, unguarded high places, areas prone to wetness and spills, and areas where clutter accumulates. The following tips will assist in the prevention of slips/trips/falls:

- Clean spills immediately.
- Put up appropriate signage where floors have been recently mopped to alert health care personnel and visitors to the danger.
- Avoid throw rugs; use nonskid rugs instead to prevent slippage.
- Be aware of cords, whether phone cords or otherwise, to prevent a trip hazard.
- Close cabinet and other doors when done.
- Do not stand on a surface that has wheels underneath.
- Maintain an uncluttered environment.

Safety Signs, Symbols, Labels

In a health care environment, it is imperative that appropriate signs be hung in areas where any potential hazards or dangers may lie to keep people safe. Knowing what common safety signs, symbols, and labels look like will help the CMA safely navigate through their environment. Commonly seen signs include the following categories:

Wet floor sign: This sign will be placed by housekeeping most commonly after mopping a floor to warn of a slip hazard.

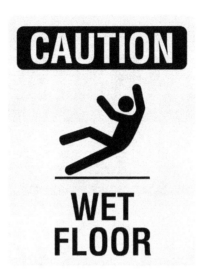

No smoking sign: Most health care facilities are smoke-free areas, so the no smoking sign will be something the CMA will be familiar with.

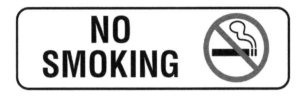

Caution: A caution sign warns of a potential hazard. This hazard may pose the risk of a minor to moderate injury to the health care worker. Caution signs are usually yellow and black.

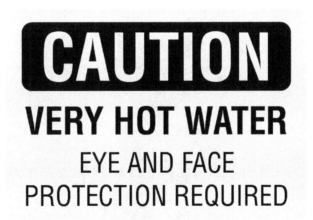

Warning: In between caution and danger signs are warning signs, indicating the potential for serious injury or even death. These signs are usually formatted as black letters on an orange background.

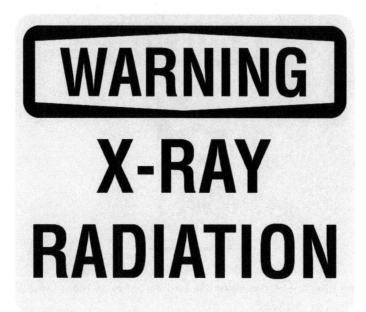

Biological hazard: This type of hazard originates in a living thing, such as bacteria, viruses, or insects.

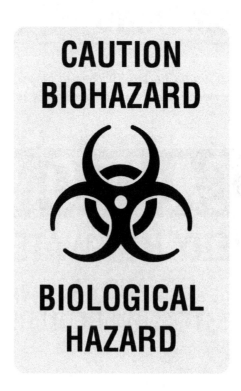

Danger: This type of safety sign indicates an immediate hazard that could cause death or serious injury.

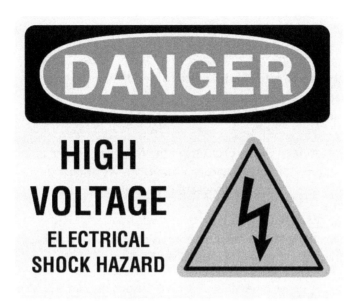

Environmental Safety

<u>Ergonomics</u>
Ergonomics studies people in their work environments and how work is most efficiently performed. It is commonly used to refer to safe lifting techniques. Health care workers are especially prone to back and knee injuries because of improper lifting techniques or too much lifting when assisting patients who cannot lift their own weight. The proper lifting technique involves the following: bending at the hips and knees, not at the back; avoiding awkward positions or twisting when lifting; holding the load as close to the body as possible; keeping a wide base of support; and always maintaining good posture.

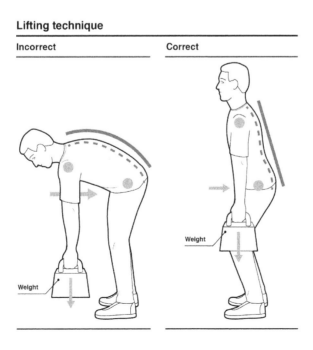

Electrical Safety

An electrical injury can cause burns, shock, and worst of all, death by electrocution. The CMA must be careful to avoid electrical hazards in their work environment, as well as working to prevent hazardous situations to patients and coworkers. The following tips will ensure electrical safety in the health care environment:

- Inspect electrical wires or cords for fraying or other damage before use.
- Tape cords to walls or floors when necessary.
- Keep electricity and water separated at all times; electricity and water do not mix, as water is a superconductor.
- Be aware of the location of circuit breakers in the facility in case of an emergency.
- Do not touch a person after an electrical accident; always disconnect the source of power and contact emergency services before proceeding to avoid electrocution.

Fire Prevention/Extinguisher Use/Regulations

All health care workers, including CMAs, must have a basic amount of training in fire safety and prevention. The basic concepts of fire safety include the following:

Fire hazards: Cigarette or any other type of smoking is a serious fire hazard. Most health care facilities are smoke-free, but some have designated areas where smoking is allowed. Patients on supplemental oxygen should not be allowed to smoke, as oxygen is highly flammable. Faulty or improperly used equipment could pose a fire hazard. The CMA should keep a lookout for frayed wires, split cords, or overloaded extension cords, as these all pose a fire hazard.

Responding to a fire: The CMA should know the facilities' procedure for responding to a fire, including the emergency plan; location of fire alarms, fire extinguishers, and emergency oxygen shutoff valves; and how to move the patients and staff to safety using emergency exits.

RACE: The acronym "RACE" refers to the following steps to be taken when responding to a fire in a health care facility:

- R: Rescue anyone directly threatened by the fire, patients being the priority, placing them in a nearby room behind a closed door.

- A: Activate the emergency response system when a fire is discovered, usually by pulling the emergency fire alarms.

- C: Confine the fire by closing all facility doors.

- E: Extinguish the fire only if it is small enough for an extinguisher to handle; otherwise, let the fire department handle it.

Fire extinguisher use: Every health care employee needs to know how to operate a fire extinguisher using the "PASS" acronym:

- P: Pull the pin.
- A: Aim at the base of the fire.
- S: Squeeze the trigger.
- S: Sweep side to side.

Compliance Reporting

Compliance means to conform to a certain rule; in health care, this usually refers to either the patients complying with their recommended plan of care and treatment or a hospital complying with state and federal standards of care. The CMA, as part of the health care team, is a mandated reporter of any health care noncompliance to the appropriate governing bodies.

Reporting Unsafe Activities and Behaviors
The CMA may witness a colleague participating in an unsafe behavior such as substance abuse. Health care workers are especially prone to substance abuse due to the high-stress work environment and relatively easy access to painkillers and other prescription drugs. It may be conflicting and feel like a betrayal, but a CMA must report this type of behavior to a supervisor. Substance abuse not only is part of a dangerous addiction, but it also poses a serious threat to patient safety.

Disclosing Errors in Patient Care
Errors are an unfortunate reality in health care, some more serious than others. A CMA or other member of the health care team that has committed an error, whether with medication administration or otherwise, may wish to conceal the error and not disclose it to anyone. Reporting an error, however embarrassing it might be, is vital to fixing an imperfect system. Health care workers might fear punitive action, but more and more organizations are moving away from this and looking for more constructive solutions. If errors are not reported, the bigger picture of how and why they occur cannot be addressed. Improvement to patient care cannot be made without error reporting.

Insurance Fraud, Waste, and Abuse
The health insurance system is unfortunately prone to fraud, waste, and abuse by its users. Fraud means an individual knowingly deceives a health benefit program to obtain said benefits. Waste entails an overuse of services that results in unnecessary costs to the system. Abuse occurs when a patient misrepresents the facts of their case to obtain payment for services for which they were not legally entitled. The CMA is to be aware of fraud, waste, and abuse as it applies to their patient population and report any suspected cases to the proper authorities.

Conflicts of Interest
Any conflict of interest witnessed by the CMA in their facility needs to be reported to the appropriate supervisor. This could include doing clinical research on a product while receiving funding from the product's owners, giving preferential treatment to a certain pharmaceutical brand or medical equipment company, accepting gifts from vendors, or owning stock in a company upon whose product one is performing clinical research, among many others.

Incident Reports
Incident reporting is a way in which patient safety can be monitored in health care systems. The CMA can voluntarily report any event involving patient safety, recording what circumstances surrounded the event, actions that led up to the event, and what took place after the incident occurred. An example of an incident report is a patient fall report. Patient falls are, unfortunately, a common occurrence in the health care environment. This type of incident report is a way to look at the fall and look for ways to prevent it from happening in the future. A drawback to incident reporting is their subjective nature, prone to bias and a limited point of view.

Medical Terminology

Part of the training of a CMA includes a course in medical terminology, a language unto itself. This language involves Latin- and Greek-derived terms for body parts, diseases, and pathologies; human anatomy and physiology terms; and procedure names. All this terminology will become second nature to the CMA as they study them and hear them in their practice.

Word Parts

Knowing the basic structure of a word, including its root, prefix, and suffix, will give the CMA the clues they need to determine the word's meaning. Many medical terms originate from Greek or Latin words.

Basic Structure
Roots/Combining Forms
A word's root, or its combining form, is the most basic part of the word. A prefix or suffix may be added to change the meaning of the word. Common root words in medical terminology and what they refer to include:

- acous- hearing
- adip- fat
- angi- cardiovascular
- bronch- bronchus
- cerebr- cerebrum
- cyst- bladder
- derma- skin
- enceph- brain
- enter- intestine
- femor- thigh bone
- gastr- stomach
- hepat- liver
- hyster- uterus
- lact- milk
- laryng- larynx
- mamm- breast
- my- muscle
- nephr- kidney
- ocul- eye
- oste- bone
- ot- ear
- pancreat- pancreas
- pneum- air, lung
- ren- kidney
- retin- retina
- somat- body
- splen- spleen
- thrombo- clot
- tympan- eardrum

- ven- vein
- vesic- bladder

Prefixes

A prefix is a group of letters that can be added to the beginning of a word to alter its meaning. The following is a list of common prefixes in medical terminology and their meanings:

- a/an- without, not, such as analgesic
- ab- from, away from, such as abnormal
- ante- before, in front of
- anti- opposing
- bi- double, two, twice, both
- co- together, with
- di- twice, two
- extro/extra- beyond, outside of, outward
- hemi- half
- hyper- above, excessive, beyond
- infra- below, beneath
- inter- between
- macro- large
- micro- small
- post- after, following, behind
- pre/pro- in front of, before, preceding
- semi- half
- trans- through, across
- tri- three
- ultra- excessive, beyond

Suffixes

The opposite of a prefix is a suffix. The suffix is the group of letters attached to the end of a root word that alters its meaning. The following is a list of common medical suffixes and their meanings:

- -ac: pertaining to, such as cardiac
- -al: pertaining to, such as abdominal
- -alge: pain, such as myalgia, a term for muscle pain
- -ate, -ize: subject to, use
- -ent, -er, -ist: person, agent
- -genic: produced by
- -gram: written record
- -graph: instrument used to record
- -graphy: process of recording
- -ism: condition or theory
- -itis: inflammation
- -ologist: one who studies, specialist
- -ology: study of, process of study
- -oma: tumor
- -pathy: disease, disease process

- -phobia: morbid fear of, intolerance
- -scope: instrument used to do a visual examination
- -scopy: process by which an exam is performed visually

Definitions/Medical Terminology

The following is a list of some common diseases, pathologies, diagnostic procedures, surgical procedures, and medical specialties that a CMA will encounter in their practice:

<u>Diseases and Pathologies</u>
- Abdominal aortic aneurysm (AAA): An aneurysm is a balloon-like bulge that can develop in a weakened wall of a blood vessel. An AAA is an aneurysm that has developed in the abdominal aorta and is a life-threatening condition. If an aneurysm bursts, the patient could hemorrhage internally and die within a matter of minutes.

- Aphasia: inability to speak or understand speech

- Apnea: the absence of breathing

- Alopecia: loss of hair

- Dysphagia: difficulty eating

- Amenorrhea: an absence of menses for a woman

- Bradycardia: slowing of the heartbeat, usually below 60 beats per minute

- Bradypnea: a decreased rate of breathing, below 12 breaths a minute

- Clostridium difficile infection: a highly contagious bacterial infection causing watery diarrhea that can result from overuse of antibiotics; a common hospital-acquired infection (HAI)

- Dyspnea: difficulty breathing

- Colitis: an inflammation of the colon characterized by diarrhea and lower abdominal pain

- Diplopia: double vision

- Hemiplegia: paralysis of one side of the body

- Gigantism: a condition in which the body oversecretes human growth hormone (HGH), resulting in a greater than normal size and height

- Menses: the time during a woman's menstrual cycle in which the uterine lining is shed; commonly called "a period"

- Lordosis: an inward curvature of the lower back, causing the abdomen to protrude; common in pregnant women

- Osteoporosis: a condition in which calcium deposits are depleted over time, weakening the bones and putting the patient at risk for fractures

- Rhinorrhea: nasal drainage or "a runny nose"

- Gynecomastia: a hormonal imbalance in males that causes an enlargement of the male breast tissue

- Rhinitis: an inflammation of the nasal tissue characterized by nasal congestion, nasal drainage, sneezing, coughing, and watery eyes

- Tachycardia: an elevated heart rate, usually above 100 beats per minute

- Tachypnea: an elevated rate of breathing, greater than 25 breaths per minute

- Urticaria: an itchy skin rash triggered by an allergic reaction; commonly called "hives"

Diagnostic Procedures
- X-ray: a test using a high-energy electromagnetic wave to visualize internal structures of the human body; useful for diagnosing broken bones and respiratory conditions such as pneumonia

- Mammography: a visualization of the breast tissue to screen for abnormalities, such as cancerous tumors

- Complete blood count: Obtained from a blood sample, this test measures the amount of red blood cells, white blood cells, and hemoglobin and can be used to diagnose various medical conditions such as anemia, leukemia, and the presence of an infection.

- Prothrombin Time (PT test): This blood test measures the amount of time it takes a patient's blood to clot and can help determine the effectiveness of blood-thinning medicine such as warfarin.

- Magnetic Resonance Imaging (MRI): This diagnostic tool gives practitioners an image of the inside of the body, like an x-ray, but with much more detail.

- Computer Axial Tomography (CT/CAT scan): a radiological diagnostic tool that can use contrast or not to produce images of the inside of the body; useful for visualization of fractures, kidney stones, tumors, and many other uses

- Echocardiography (ECHO): a type of ultrasound that visualizes the chambers of the heart as well as surrounding structures; used to diagnose heart conditions and evaluate overall function

- Colonoscopy: a visualization, using a "scope" or tiny camera at the end of a long tube, of the colon; most often used to screen for colorectal cancer, remove polyps, and diagnose other colonic conditions

- Bone density study: a test like an x-ray that is used to visualize bones and assess bone loss

- Prostate-Specific Antigen (PSA): This test is used to screen for prostate cancer or other diseases of the male prostate gland; an elevation could indicate a pathology is at work.

- Electrocardiogram (EKG or ECG): A test in which electrodes placed on the patient's chest pick up the electrical activity of the heart; abnormalities can be detected using this noninvasive test, such as heart dysrhythmias and myocardial damage.

- Bronchoscopy: a visualization of the internal passages of the lung, usually performed by a pulmonologist, using a long tube with a camera at the end called a "scope"; used for tissue sampling or biopsy and to diagnose conditions such as lung cancer

Surgical Procedures
- Mastectomy: removal of a part of the breast or the entire breast; used for treating breast cancer

- Hysterectomy: removal of a woman's uterus, potentially for uterine cancer, fibroids, or endometriosis, among other reasons

- Dilation and curettage (D&C): procedure where a woman's cervix is dilated and the uterine lining is scraped out using a spoon-like device called a *curette*; used for elective abortions, miscarriages, and any other time the contents of the uterus need to be evacuated

- Carotid endarterectomy: procedure in which blockages are removed from the carotid arteries located in the neck, usually for prevention of stroke

- Breast biopsy: removal of breast tissue, usually a lump, to screen for cancer and other conditions

- Appendectomy: removal of the appendix in the treatment of appendicitis, an inflammation of the appendix

- Cataract surgery: removal of cataracts from the lens of the eye using ultrasound waves, sometimes involving the removal of the entire lens depending on the severity of the disease

- Cholecystectomy: removal of the gall bladder; can be for a cancerous gall bladder, one prone to gallstones, or infection

- Cesarean section (C-section): delivery of a baby through a lower abdominal incision when vaginal delivery is deemed an unsafe option; can be an elective or emergent procedure

- Coronary artery bypass (CABG) surgery: also known as open-heart surgery, a procedure in which the patient's chest is opened at the sternum and grafting of leg veins is performed to repair or bypass clogged or narrowed arteries supplying the cardiac muscle with blood; for patients with a history of atherosclerotic disease

- Wound debridement: removal of dead tissue from a wound to promote healing

Medical Specialties
- Pulmonologist: lung doctor

- Cardiologist: heart doctor

- Immunologist: doctor who specializes in the care of immune conditions

- Cardiovascular surgeon: doctor who specializes in surgical procedures on the heart and its structures, as well as performing procedures involving the circulatory system

- Geriatric medicine specialist: doctor who specializes in treating an older, or geriatric, population

- Hepatologist: doctor specializing in the treatment of hepatic conditions, or conditions of the liver

- Nephrologist: doctor who specializes in the treatment of renal or kidney conditions

- Internist: doctor who practices internal medicine, meaning they work within a hospital, treating patients who have been hospitalized, rather than having an office and working with outpatients; also called *hospitalists*

- Gastroenterologist: doctor who specializes in the treatment of GI conditions

- Hematologist: doctor who specializes in the treatment of blood disorders

- Obstetrician: doctor who specializes in treating women who are pregnant; practices obstetrics

- Gynecologist: doctor who specializes in women's health, as well as diagnosing and treating diseases of the female reproductive system

- Oncologist: doctor who specializes in cancer treatment

- Ophthalmologist: doctor who specializes in eye health

- Ear-Nose-Throat (ENT): doctor who specializes in the ear-nose-throat health; also called an *otolaryngologist*

Practice Questions

1. According to Maslow's hierarchy of needs, what is the highest level on the pyramid?
    a. Prestige
    b. Accomplishment
    c. Self-esteem
    d. Self-actualization

2. At the end of one's life, what virtue does Erikson's stages of development say develops when one has positively overcome the ego conflict of integrity vs. despair?
    a. Fidelity
    b. Wisdom
    c. Caring
    d. Love

3. A patient is verbally abusive toward the CMA. On a follow-up visit, the same patient is overly nice to the same CMA, flattering them and complimenting them nonstop. The CMA recognizes this as which defense mechanism?
    a. Undoing
    b. Denial
    c. Sublimation
    d. Repression

4. Which of the following techniques will aid in communicating with a patient who is blind?
    a. Speaking loudly to ensure the patient can hear the message
    b. Using hand gestures to aid in conveying the message
    c. Turning off the TV to decrease distractions
    d. Speaking slowly so the patient can keep up with the message

5. The CMA is assessing the patient's level of understanding preceding a complicated procedure. The patient explains their impression of what will happen, and the CMA paraphrases what the patient says back to them. What type of technique did the CMA employ here?
    a. Restatement
    b. Reflection
    c. Clarification
    d. Feedback

6. The CMA is attempting to gather some information from the patient for a health history, but the patient appears to be grimacing, uncomfortable, and distracted. What type of distraction is the patient likely experiencing?
    a. Pain
    b. Noise
    c. Disinterest
    d. Temperature

7. The CMA is conducting a patient interview to gather a health history. The CMA asks the patient if she has taken her blood pressure medicine today. This is an example of which type of information-gathering question?
    a. Exploratory
    b. Rhetorical
    c. Open-ended
    d. Closed

8. A CMA should try and present a professional image through all but which of the following?
    a. Come to work wearing the appropriate uniform and grooming appropriately.
    b. Speak to patients with care and courtesy.
    c. Take part in volunteer events to help the poor and needy in the community.
    d. Post pictures to social media of the workplace, and post status updates talking about work gossip.

9. The Health Insurance Portability Accountability Act (HIPAA) was enacted for all but which of the following reasons?
    a. Decrease inefficiencies and reduce paperwork within the health insurance system.
    b. Ensure that the testing of human laboratory specimens meets federal standards.
    c. Prevent duplication of services through coordination of care.
    d. Protect patient health information privacy and confidentiality.

10. A CMA is taking care of a patient who has been incapacitated by a severe stroke two years ago. The patient's daughter makes her health care decisions for her legally through which specific legal document?
    a. Medical durable power of attorney
    b. Living will
    c. Advance directives
    d. Patient Self-Determination Act

11. The CMA knows that marijuana, though legalized and used medically in many states, is still listed by the Drug Enforcement Agency (DEA) as a Schedule I drug, meaning which of the following?
    a. No potential for abuse
    b. Low potential for abuse
    c. Moderate potential for abuse
    d. High potential for abuse

12. The CMA protects patient privacy and confidentiality according to which law?
    a. Genetic Information Nondiscrimination Act of 2008
    b. Health Information Technology for Economic and Clinical Act
    c. Health Insurance Portability and Accountability Act
    d. Public Health and Welfare Disclosure

13. The doctor has just finished explaining a procedure to a patient and answering their questions. The patient seems to understand and has signed a document stating they are permitting the procedure to be done and that they understand the side effects and potential complications. What type of consent was obtained?
   a. Expressed consent
   b. Informed consent
   c. Implied consent
   d. Verbal consent

14. Which of the following Latin phrases means "let the master answer" and means that the employer is legally responsible for the actions of their employees?
   a. Subpoena duces tecum
   b. Res ipsa loquitur
   c. Locum tenens
   d. Respondeat superior

15. What type of law is based on previously decided court cases, or precedents?
   a. Common
   b. Civil
   c. Criminal
   d. Statutory

16. The CMA is taking care of a patient who has recently been diagnosed with a terminal cancer. It is looking like the disease will take a long time to take its course, and the patient has talked about euthanasia as an option. The CMA knows that which of the following is false regarding euthanasia?
   a. Euthanasia is an ethical gray area with which the CMA may not agree.
   b. Euthanasia is sometimes called "physician-assisted suicide" or "death with dignity."
   c. Euthanasia allows a patient to die on their own terms rather than having a lot of potential pain and suffering with a drawn-out disease.
   d. Euthanasia is illegal in all 50 states of the United States.

17. A CMA suspects that a physician he works for has been abusing painkillers. The physician has been coming to work seemingly under the influence, slurring his speech and more clumsy than usual. The CMA knows that he is going through a divorce, and it has been causing him extra stress. Normally, the physician is completely competent and has a good rapport with his patients. What should the CMA do, since the physician is his supervisor?
   a. Tell his fellow CMAs what he thinks but not take it any further.
   b. Wait until there is more solid evidence, such as a medication or prescription error.
   c. Report his suspicions to the appropriate supervising body, such as human resources.
   d. Keep an eye on the physician for the next couple months; maybe after the divorce is completed, he will quit taking the painkillers.

18. The CMA is preparing to take the vital signs of a patient with an electronic blood pressure machine. The CMA notices that the wires are frayed on the electrical cord of the machine. What is an appropriate action that the CMA should take when seeing this?

    a. Proceed with taking the blood pressure.

    b. Try using a different electrical outlet to plug the cord into.

    c. Attempt to repair the cord by wrapping some medical tape around it.

    d. Report the issue to maintenance or whoever maintains equipment in the CMA's facility; look for a different blood pressure machine to take the reading with or check the blood pressure manually.

19. A CMA is assisting a patient from the bed to his wheelchair. When using proper lifting technique, which of the following is incorrect?

    a. Bend at the knees, and lift with the legs.

    b. Maintain a wide base of support for maximum strength.

    c. Keep the patient load an arm's length away from the body for infection prevention.

    d. Maintain proper and erect posture.

20. A fire alarm has been pulled in the office building where the CMA works. Which of the following steps of the RACE acronym will help contain a fire?

    a. Close all facility doors, including patient room doors.

    b. Remove clutter from the hallway to ensure emergency exits are easily accessed.

    c. Activate the emergency response system.

    d. Rescue anyone directly threatened by the fire.

21. A small fire has developed in the employee's break room of the facility. The CMA grabs the fire extinguisher and follows which of the following instructions to operate the extinguisher properly?

    a. CMAs are not authorized to use fire extinguishers. The CMA should find an authorized member of the team to use the extinguisher.

    b. Aim at the middle of the fire, pull the pin, and sweep from side to side while squeezing the trigger.

    c. Squeeze the trigger, aim at the top of the flames, and sweep up and down until the flames are extinguished.

    d. Pull the pin, aim at the base of the fire, squeeze the trigger, and sweep from side to side until the fire is extinguished.

22. The CMA has taken the patient's vital signs and notes her to be "bradycardic." What does this mean?

    a. Her blood pressure is less than 90 systolic and 60 diastolic.

    b. Her rate of breathing is less than 12 breaths per minute.

    c. Her heart rate is less than 60 beats per minute.

    d. Her bowel sounds are occurring less than 5 times per minute.

23. A patient has a history of chest pain and was recently hospitalized for a myocardial infarction, or heart attack. The patient is now an outpatient seeing his cardiologist for a follow-up evaluation. The CMA is asked to perform a procedure to assess the electrical rhythm of the patient's heart known as which of the following?

    a. ECG

    b. ECHO

    c. EFG

    d. EEG

24. The CMA is taking care of a patient who has been advised to have a carotid endarterectomy. The CMA knows that this procedure is done to prevent which life-threatening condition?
   a. Myocardial infarction
   b. Pulmonary embolism
   c. Stroke
   d. Hyperthyroidism

25. Which of the following refers to a doctor who specializes in treating blood disorders such as sickle cell anemia?
   a. Hepatologist
   b. Hematologist
   c. Cardiologist
   d. Immunology

26. Which of the following is NOT an element of informed consent for a surgical procedure?
   a. A detailed explanation of the planned procedure
   b. Identification of all reasonable alternative options
   c. Waiver of injury compensation
   d. Discussion of possible complications that may occur if the procedure is not performed

27. As a healthcare provider, the CMA must understand the limits of the Good Samaritan Law. Which of the following statements is consistent with this law?
   a. All individuals that provide emergency care are protected by the law.
   b. The Good Samaritan Law is a federal law that has been ratified by all states.
   c. Providers are protected from legal action.
   d. Trained health care providers are covered for emergency care delivered in their place of employment.

28. Which of the following activities is within the scope of practice of the CMA?
   a. Collecting blood and urine specimens for analysis
   b. Creating a teaching plan for a newly prescribed medication
   c. Explaining the results of the A1C to a patient
   d. Evaluating the patient's compliance with the plan of care

Answer Explanations

1. D: The highest level of Maslow's hierarchy of needs is self-actualization, in which one achieves their full potential, including creative pursuits. Prestige, a feeling of accomplishment, and self-esteem are all part of the esteem needs, one level below the top and part of the psychological needs section.

2. B: Wisdom is the virtue that is developed if the ego conflict of integrity vs. despair is positively overcome. Fidelity is the virtue that comes after identity vs. role confusion is positively overcome. Caring is the virtue that is developed after the ego conflict of generativity vs. stagnation is positively overcome. Love is the virtue that comes out of a positive outcome of the intimacy vs. isolation conflict.

3. A: The patient is demonstrating "undoing"—a defense mechanism that attempts to undo a wrong or bad action with the opposite action. Denial is a defense mechanism in which a person simply denies a reality because they do not want to deal with potentially painful emotions. Sublimation is a defense mechanism in which negative impulses are channeled into positive action. Repression is a defense mechanism in which a person unconsciously avoids thoughts about something painful, similar to the conscious act of suppression.

4. C: Turning off the TV in a patient's room always helps with clear communication. If a patient is blind, the CMA should not treat them as if they are hard of hearing or have an intellectual deficit by speaking loudly or slowly. Using hand gestures is useless if the patient is blind.

5. B: By paraphrasing what the patient says, the CMA is using the reflection technique to assess the patient's level of understanding. Restatement means to repeat exactly what the patient says back to them. Clarification involves questions and repeating back the essential meaning to the patient. Feedback involves more of a reaction to what the patient says with a desire to improve the relationship and further communications.

6. A: The patient appears to be experiencing the internal distraction of pain. Noise and temperature are examples of external distractions that create a barrier to communication and information gathering. Disinterest is a barrier to communication that would present itself differently from pain, in ways such as yawning, lack of eye contact, and slouching.

7. C: This question can be answered with a "yes" or a "no," so it is a closed question. An exploratory question is a specific type of open-ended question in which a subject is dissected and investigated in depth. A rhetorical question is one that is asked that does not require any answer at all; it is simply asked for the sake of being asked. An example of a rhetorical answer would be, "Is it ever going to stop raining?" The person asking logically knows that the rain always stops eventually. They are venting their frustration about the rain and impatience for better weather by asking a rhetorical question. Open-ended questions require the person to give a more detailed answer than just "yes" or "no." An example would be asking the patient what they are feeling, inviting a descriptive and detailed answer.

8. D: The CMA must maintain a professional image, as they are a representative of a respected profession: medical assisting. Posting gossip-type information as well as photos that could violate HIPAA contribute to an unprofessional—not to mention immature—image of CMAs and should be avoided. The consequences could be serious for the CMA as far as their employment and ability to practice are concerned.

9. B: HIPAA was enacted to protect patient privacy and confidentiality as well as to decrease inefficiencies and reduce paperwork to speed up the claims process. Human laboratory specimens meeting federal standards is part of the Clinical Laboratory Improvement Act (CLIA) of 1988.

10. A: The specific document that appoints a person (usually a family member) to make medical decisions for a patient when they become incapacitated is the medical durable power of attorney. The power of attorney can be part of both the living will and advance directives in general. The difference is that a living will (Choice *B*) is a broader document that covers many topics regarding a patient's care, such as if they would ever want a feeding tube should they become unable to feed themselves and/or eat. Advance directives, Choice *C*, is an even broader category covering both living wills and powers of attorney. All patients should be encouraged to draw up advance directive documents. Choice *D*, Patient Self-Determination Act, is the act that requires facilities to give patients certain documents upon arrival and states that facilities cannot discriminate against patients who have or do not have an advanced directive.

11. D: Schedule I drugs, according to the DEA, have a high potential for abuse and have no accepted safety for use under medical supervision, even though some states have legalized their use for medicinal and recreational reasons. Other Schedule I drugs include heroin, LSD, ecstasy, and bath salts. Schedule II drugs also have a high potential for abuse but have medically accepted reasons for use, at least according to the DEA.

12. C: A patient's health information is to remain private and confidential, according to the Health Insurance Portability and Accountability Act, commonly known as HIPAA. The other three items listed, Genetic Information Nondiscrimination Act (GINA) of 2008, Health Information Technology for Economic and Clinical Health (HITECH), and Public Health and Welfare Disclosure, do not have to do exclusively with patient privacy. HITECH involves patient access to their own medical record, GINA was enacted to prevent patients from being discriminated against based on their genetics, and Public Health and Welfare Disclosure has to do with disease prevention within a population.

13. B: When a patient has been adequately informed about a procedure or decision and signs a document granting their permission to commence, it is called *informed consent*. Expressed or verbal consent is when the patient consents merely with a gesture such as a nod or verbally agrees. Implied consent is when there is not necessarily any formal agreement made verbally, through gestures or through writing, but consent is assumed. Usually, implied consent is used in emergency situations or for small, minor procedures.

14. D: *Respondeat superior* comes from the Latin words that mean "let the master answer" and means that an employer is legally responsible for the actions of their employee. *Subpoena duces tecum* means "under penalty you shall bring with you" and means that a person must come to court with any pertinent evidence. *Res ipsa loquitur* translates from Latin as "the thing speaks for itself" and indicates that negligence can be blamed when an accident happens. *Locum tenens* is Latin for "one holding a place" and is used when a physician is filling in for another.

15. A: Common law is based on precedents, or previously decided court cases. Civil law involves disputes between individuals and community members. Criminal law involves consequences for those who commit crimes. Statutory law is based on laws passed through legislative action.

16. D: Euthanasia is now legal in a few states in the United States. The other three statements are true. It is an ethical gray area and an issue that may become more prevalent in the coming years as it potentially becomes legalized. It is called "death with dignity" and "physician-assisted suicide" and is a way to bypass potential pain and suffering. The CMA needs to be aware of this ethical issue in their practice.

17. C: The CMA should report his suspicion of substance abuse to HR. Even if he is wrong about the substance abuse, ethically it is the right thing to do. Gossiping to fellow employees does nothing and could be more damaging. Ignoring it and/or not doing anything about it could result in serious patient harm, and the CMA may be named in the case if any litigation were to arise out of the matter. Substance abusers need help with stress and addiction management. By reporting and addressing the problem of substance abuse, those who are addicted can find help to overcoming their addiction.

18. D: Reporting the issue and obtaining the blood pressure reading via a different machine or manually would be the most appropriate action for the CMA to take. Not doing anything about it could lead to patient or CMA harm. Using a different outlet would not fix the problem. The fraying of the wires presents an electrocution and/or a fire hazard that needs to be addressed.

19. C: When lifting, proper technique dictates that the load be kept close to the body. Infection prevention requires appropriate personal protective equipment (PPE) if that is a concern. The other three items listed (bending at knees and lifting with legs, wide base, proper posture) are all part of proper lifting technique.

20. A: Closing all the facility doors will help confine the fire. The hallways should always remain uncluttered and emergency exits unblocked for general workplace safety. Activating the emergency response system and rescuing patients are part of the RACE acronym but will not directly affect the confinement of the fire.

21. D: The CMA should follow the "PASS" acronym for proper use of a fire extinguisher: Pull the pin, aim at the base of the fire, squeeze the trigger, and sweep from side to side until the flames are extinguished. CMAs are, in fact, authorized to use extinguishers, and finding someone else to do it would waste precious time that could be used to extinguish the fire. The other directions have elements of the "PASS" acronym but are not in the right order or worded correctly.

22. C: The patient is bradycardic when their heart rate is less than 60 beats per minute. Hypotension is a reading of less than 90 systolic and 60 diastolic. Bradypnea is a rate of breaths less than 12 breaths per minute. When a patient's bowel sounds do not occur more than 5 times per minute, it is referred to as having decreased bowel sounds.

23. A: An ECG or EKG, short for electrocardiogram, is a test using electrodes attached to the patient's chest to assess electrical activity of the heart. An echocardiogram, or ECHO, is a test using ultrasound waves to visualize the heart and its chambers to assess heart function. EFG is not a medical test. An EEG, or electroencephalogram, is used to measure and assess the electrical activity of the brain.

24. C: A carotid endarterectomy is often performed in patients with clogged or narrowed carotid arteries to prevent a stroke from a dislodged clot. Myocardial infarction, or a heart attack, can happen as a result of a clot but is not the biggest concern with atherosclerotic carotid arteries, which are very close to the brain where strokes occur. A pulmonary embolism is another condition involving clots but also is not the greatest concern directly related to carotid arteries. Though the carotid arteries are located in the neck, similar to the thyroid gland, they do not have anything to do with hyperthyroidism.

25. B: A hematologist is a doctor who specializes in the diagnosis and treatment of hematological or blood disorders such as sickle cell anemia. A hepatologist specializes in hepatic or liver disorders. A cardiologist deals with the heart and cardiovascular system but not specifically blood disorders. An immunologist takes care of disorders of the immune system, which involves the white blood cells of the blood but is not blood-specific.

26. C: Patients are not required to waive possible compensation for possible injuries. Informed consent forms should not include any waiver of the patient's rights. The remainder of the choices, Choices *A, B,* and *D,* are essential elements of informed consent and therefore are incorrect.

27. C: In many states, trained health care providers are not protected from legal action if they render care. The CMA must be aware of all applicable state laws. In some states, health care workers are the only class of individuals covered by the law, therefore, Choice *A* is incorrect. The law is a state law rather than a federal law, and while the general intent of the law is common among states, health care providers must understand the details of the law in their practice location, therefore, Choice *B* is incorrect. Trained providers are not covered for emergency care in their place of employment; therefore, Choice *D* is incorrect.

28. A: Collecting laboratory specimens for analysis is an activity that is within the scope of practice of the CMA. Evaluation, interpretation of results and constructing elements of the plan of care all require the expertise of licensed providers including physicians and nurses. Therefore, Choices *B, C,* and *D* are incorrect.

Administrative

Medical Reception

Medical Record Preparation

The certified medical assistant (CMA) understands that the medical record is a legal document that is unique to the individual patient. The medical record is prepared and maintained by all providers who render care to the patient. Depending on contracted responsibilities, the CMA may assemble the necessary components of a blank record, or they may provide and document patient care in the medical record.

Although there are government incentives for primary care agencies to implement electronic health records (EHRs), those programs are temporary, and approximately 20% of providers have not yet implemented EHRs. The CMA must be aware that all software interfaces for the EHR require training and continuing education to ensure the accuracy of the documents. In addition, all providers are required to be prepared to transfer an electronic copy of the EHR to another provider or agency upon receipt of a written request from a patient or the patient's representative. Individual requests for copies of EHRs must be satisfied within thirty days, unless there is satisfactory evidence of a reason for a one-time 30-day extension. The CMA understands and complies with all agency policies related to the confidential transfer of documents.

If the CMA is responsible for paper documents, the CMA recognizes that, as a legal document, the medical record must be accurate, complete, legible, and arranged in a logical order per agency policy. The CMA verifies that any corrections to the document are noted in the accepted manner: the entire original entry must be legible, struck with a single line, and signed with the provider's name and the date of the correction.

Demographic Data Review

The CMA understands that the required demographic data associated with the medical record includes the patient's preferred language, gender, race, ethnicity, and date of birth. If a patient declines to provide any of this data, or if the recording of any of this data is prohibited by state law, the CMA is required to include that circumstance in the health record per agency policy.

Identify Theft Protection
Providers are required to make all reasonable efforts to protect privileged health information (PHI) from cyber-security breaches by outside sources. In addition, the CMA must comply with all agency protocols that are designed to minimize the risk of identity theft in the form of insurance fraud whereby an individual misuses the identity of another person to access care. The CMA may be responsible for adding a patient's photograph to the EHR, verifying the patient's picture ID upon arrival at the agency, or participating in routine audits of financial data.

Insurance Eligibility Verification
To verify insurance coverage, the CMA retrieves the patient's demographic and insurance data from the EHR, and then contacts the insurance provider to verify coverage for the intended date of service, identifies the amount of any co-pay or costs not covered by the policy, and verifies any deductible. If

there are costs not covered by the policy, the CMA should notify the patient prior the agency appointment.

Handling Vendors or Business Associates

The CMA maintains a professional demeanor and appearance at all times while interacting with various business interests that support the work of the providers.

Reception Room Environment

Comfort
Providers ensure that the reception area is large enough to accommodate the expected number of patients. Furniture in the seating area should be comfortable and appropriate to the needs of the patient population served by the agency.

Safety
The reception room must be accessible. It must also have appropriate environmental control, and careful attention should be paid to the maintenance of all facilities and furnishings.

Sanitation
The CMA understands that the sanitation of the reception room must be a priority for aesthetic purposes as well as infection control purposes. All surfaces and furnishings must be cleaned with approved cleaning agents per agency protocol. In addition to regularly scheduled maintenance, the providers ensure that there are resources in place to respond immediately to any incident that may occur in the reception area.

Practice Information Packet

Office Policies
The provider establishes office policies and coordinates the development of patient information documents with the CMA. The CMA verifies that each patient receives all necessary information relative to policies concerning appointments, communication, insurance coverage, in addition to an introduction to agency providers and staff.

Patient Financial Responsibilities
As part of the agency admission process, the CMA verifies the terms of the patient's insurance coverage; however, the patient is ultimately responsible for verifying and complying with the terms of that coverage. The patient is responsible for co-pays due at the time of the appointment in addition to any out-of-network fees or uncovered costs.

Patient Navigator and Advocate

Resource Information

Provide Information About Community Resources
The CMA provides patients with information about the services provided by community resources, as directed by the provider. These resources may include home-based nursing care, physical or occupational therapy, or other forms of assistance.

<u>Facilitate Referrals to Community Resources</u>
The CMA provides the patient with the current contact information for the specific agency.

<u>Referral Follow-Up</u>
The CMA should also verify that the patient was successful in accessing the recommended community services. If the patient was not successful, the CMA intervenes on the patient's behalf to ensure that the patient receives appropriate care.

Medical Business Practices

Written Communication

<u>Letters</u>
Providers routinely send letters to patients containing explanations of recent test results, referral information, or reminders for follow-up care. The CMA prepares and sends all provider letters per agency policy.

<u>Memos and Interoffice Communications</u>
The CMA prepares and distributes all interoffice communication, ensuring that all print materials are grammatically correct and contain appropriate content.

<u>Reports</u>
The CMA participates in data collection and preparation of all reports as required by the agency. These reports may include agency financial statements, insurance reconciliation reports, and regulatory data reports. The CMA verifies that all reports are grammatically correct, accurate, and complete.

Business Equipment

<u>Routine Maintenance</u>
The CMA establishes and maintains a routine maintenance schedule for all office equipment. Maintenance includes ensuring office equipment is functioning properly and supplies such as ink cartridges and paper are always available.

<u>Safety Precautions</u>
The CMA should be familiar with all functions and related safety precautions for business equipment and should serve as a resource for agency staff.

Office Supply Inventory

<u>Inventory Control and Record Keeping</u>
The CMA participates in all agency cost-containment procedures, including participating in and reporting on inventory control. Proper inventory control contributes to cost-containment and ensures the availability of necessary resources.

Electronic Applications

<u>Medical Management Systems</u>
Medical management systems are computer software systems that manage agency functions.

- Database reports: Software modules may be used to manage billing, insurance claims processing, patient communication and reminders, EHR integration, Code Sets, appointment scheduling, patient demographics, and regulatory data collection. The CMA maintains proficiency in database management.

- Meaningful use regulations: Meaningful use refers to the government-funded financial incentive program that rewards providers for meaningful use of EHRs. This program is directed at improving patient care. Eligible providers must document specific performance benchmarks each year, and although the original meaningful use standards are under revision, the original objectives of the initiative remain in place. The CMA maintains proficiency related to the necessary data collection and documentation for each of the objectives, including: protection of all electronic health data, use of clinical algorithms for complex care decisions, computerized ordering of medications, documentation of all laboratory and radiology testing, timely transfer of patient data to alternate providers or agencies, provision of patient-specific educational resources available to the patient, timely patient access to all health information via patient portals, secured electronic messaging between providers and patients, and timely submission of all public health data. The CMA is aware that these objectives are subject to outcomes analysis, which means that the accurate documentation of patient outcomes is essential.

Spreadsheet and Graphs

The CMA maintains proficiency in interpreting and presenting data in the form of spreadsheets and graphs to accurately communicate information related to agency management.

Electronic Mail

The CMA uses the secure agency electronic mail system exclusively for agency-related communication, and refrains from conducting any personal business on the agency network. In addition, the CMA does not share passwords or gain access to any stored data that is beyond the scope of the CMA's practice. If the CMA is required to communicate with patients or other individuals outside of the agency staff, the CMA uses appropriate language, grammar, and spelling for all communication.

Security

- Password or screensaver: The CMA safeguards the agency-issued password and resets the password when prompted by the computer system. All computer screens not in use must be "dark," so that only the specified screensaver is visible.

- Encryption: The provider employs all possible safeguards to secure PHI. All agency employees use only encrypted systems to transmit PHI.

- Firewall: All agency networks should be protected by a firewall, and agency employees should not attempt to by-pass the firewall for any reason. The CMA complies with all computer safety and security standards.

Transmission of Information

- Facsimile or scanner: A government-approved cover sheet should be applied to all PHI that is sent to another agency or provider. The cover should not contain PHI beyond the patient's name and two other unique identifiers such as a medical record number or birthdate. Prior to sending the fax, the CMA collects all intended PHI for transmission, confirms the fax number for the receiving party, and communicates with the receiving party to verify that the information was received. All PHI that is electronically forwarded to other agencies or providers must be assembled logically and should contain the appropriate information.

If the scanner is used to duplicate documents for transfer, the CMA verifies that scanned copies are legible and that all original documents are removed from the scanner to avoid breaches of confidentiality and lost data.

- Patient portal to health data: The meaningful use criteria mandate the use of the patient portal to facilitate patient access to PHI. Providers are responsible for purchasing the computer platform, educating agency staff in its use, and ensuring timely posting of relevant PHI. Although many providers are looking forward to second generation software to eliminate the initial implementation difficulties, the use of the portal as a communication tool has improved patient satisfaction, and its use as a scheduling tool has decreased the number of missed appointments. Many providers contend that patients are more likely to become more involved in their own care and report feeling less isolated from their providers.

Social Media

Social media connects the agency, the providers, and the staff with the community. Social media provides unique information in an informal way that allows prospective patients to learn about the provider and the agency. The CMA maintains the currency of the information posted on the agency sites and reports patient feedback to the providers as appropriate.

Establish Patient Medical Record

Recognizing and Interpreting Data

The CMA recognizes the purpose and appropriate format for each element of the EHR, and collates all data per agency protocol.

History and Physical

The provider performs a physical examination and collects a medical history from every patient during the initial contact. This data is documented as the history and physical, and is most often the initial clinical element of the EHR.

Discharge Summary

The provider completes a discharge summary when a patient is moved from one facility to another, discharged to home, or to the care of an alternate provider. The discharge summary should include the initial presenting complaint and all subsequent PHI. The CMA verifies that the transcription is accurate and appropriately signed and dated.

Operative Note

The provider completes the operative note, which includes the details of any surgical procedure with notation of all events from the pre-anesthesia unit to the post-anesthesia unit. Depending on the agency format, the operative note should also contain the operative data from the anesthesia and nursing services.

Diagnostic Tests and Lab Reports

The CMA verifies that all diagnostic testing data, including imaging studies, laboratory tests, and pathology reports, is added to the EHR.

Clinical Progress Notes

The CMA understands that the format of the clinical progress notes is dictated by the documentation format of the providers. As noted below, the record may be a problem-oriented medical record (POMR) which means that all providers address the patient problems in chronological order in a single document. A source-oriented medical record (SOMR) contains chronological notes from each individual provider: physician's notes, nurse's notes, physical therapist's notes, and so on. The CMA understands the requirements for each format and verifies that the clinical notes are complete.

Consultation Report
The consultation report documents the patient care from an alternate provider at the request of the primary care provider (PCP). The CMA verifies that the EHR includes data from all consulting providers.

Correspondence
The CMA identifies and includes any additional correspondence related to the patient's care in the EHR. Possible sources of additional correspondence include laboratory results for outside agencies, community resource communications, and alternate provider information.

Charts, Graphs, Tables
As previously mentioned, the analysis and documentation of patient outcomes are essential elements of the primary care practice. The CMA verifies that any patient data generated in the form of charts, graphs, and tables is included in the EHR.

Flow Sheet
The patient care flow sheet is used to document chronological assessment data that most often includes vital signs, common lab values including blood glucose values, and body weight. The CMA verifies that all required documentation is included for each patient visit.

Charting Systems

POMR
The POMR documents a problem-solving approach to patient care that requires identification of a patient's health problems; documentation of the care aimed at control or resolution of those problems, from all providers; facilitation of continuing assessment of patient outcomes; and revisions of the treatment plan by all providers. The CMA maintains the POMR per agency policy in a format that is easily accessible to all providers. The initial entry to the record is the patient history, which includes the information obtained from the patient and their family during the admission interview. This information is an essential element of the patient's problem list, and it must include the history of the current concern or illness; the history of past illnesses and surgeries, including data from other providers; relevant family health history; and a subjective review of the systems.

The second major element of the record is documentation of the results of the physical examination. The CMA recognizes that the scope of that examination is determined by the patient's presenting illness or condition.

The third element of the POMR is the master problem list, which is a compilation of the problems and concerns identified in the initial patient interview and the physical examination. The individual problems may relate to physical, emotional, or socio-economic conditions or concerns. In addition, the problems are designated as active, inactive, temporary, or potential, and it is expected that these labels should be revised over time as a means of outcomes assessment. The chronological list of the patient problems is recorded in a database with a column for each of the following: the problem, the date of problem onset, the action taken, the outcome or resolution, and the date of the outcome or resolution. This format provides a flexible document that allows for the addition of new problems and the addition and revision of planned interventions that is accessible to all providers.

<u>Source-Oriented Medical Record (SOMR)</u>
The CMA understands that the SOMR contains individual entries by each provider involved the care of an individual patient. For instance, all nursing care, medical care, and physical therapy are documented in separate chronologically oriented files by the provider. The CMA collates the individual records per agency protocol.

Scheduling Appointments

Scheduling Guidelines

The CMA recognizes that appropriate scheduling significantly affects patient satisfaction. Patients expect minimal wait times during scheduling and at appointments. In order to schedule appointments appropriately, the CMA must: protect patient confidentiality in the office setting, maintain focus on one person at a time, speak clearly and repeat information for clarity, obtain all the patient information that is necessary to schedule the appropriate amount of time for the appointment, and enter the appointment details in the agency scheduling system or appointment book.

<u>Appointment Matrix</u>
The appointment matrix is the foundation of the scheduling process. The CMA first blocks the hours that the agency is closed and then blocks the hours when each of the providers is not available. The use of the matrix is guided by specific instructions from the providers regarding appropriate time allocation for specific patient encounters. For instance, the provider may require more time to be scheduled for a patient appointment for an annual physical examination than for a blood pressure check. In addition, the providers may block a period of time each day to accommodate same-day appointments for patients with acute illnesses, or as "catch up" time to allow for patient appointments that exceed the original time allotment.

<u>New Patient Appointments</u>
The new patient appointment should be scheduled for 30-45 minutes, per protocol. The CMA verifies that the patient understands the scheduling details, and the CMA informs the patient of any pre-appointment paperwork to be completed. In addition, the agency provides the patient with a welcoming package that includes the details of the agency policies, providers, and staff.

To schedule an appointment for a new patient, the CMA identifies the patient's demographic data, the reason for the requested visit, and, if applicable, the name of the referring physician. If the patient has been referred for treatment by another physician, the CMA consults with the provider for proper patient scheduling. The CMA also must be aware of insurance referral requirements for agency providers.

<u>Established Patient Appointments</u>
The CMA understands that per insurance regulations, an established patient is an individual who has been seen by an agency provider in the previous three years and has a current medical record.

- Routine: The provider identifies the time period for follow-up visits on the patient encounter form, such as six weeks, one month, or annually. The CMA schedules the follow-up visit within the requested time frame for the appropriate amount of time required for the visit. Whenever possible, the CMA accommodates the patient's request for specific appointment dates and times. The appointment entry in the database requires verification of the patient's name, date of birth, and name of the provider. The CMA also gives the patient a written reminder card for the appointment that includes the date and time of the appointment, the provider's name, and instructions for canceling the appointment.

- Urgent or emergency: The providers establish the agency protocol for scheduling urgent or emergent patient care needs which includes specific instructions for the CMA when communicating with patients who are reporting emergency conditions. The CMA recognizes that common urgent or emergent conditions that may be accommodated with same-day appointments include: muscle strains and sprains; wounds that are not accompanied by bone fracture or dislocation; episodes of nausea, vomiting, and diarrhea that persist for more than 3-4 days; sore throat, especially if associated with elevated temperature; urinary symptoms with fever or bleeding; fever greater than 101° F. in adults and 102°F.-103°F. in children, and any other illness or severe pain without bleeding, fainting, or loss of consciousness.

- Critical conditions: The CMA knows critical conditions must be referred immediately to emergency medical services. The CMA recognizes that these critical conditions include: respiratory distress or arrest; chest pain or cardiac arrest; uncontrolled bleeding; large, open wounds; symptoms that are associated with internal bleeding; potential poisoning or overdose; any abnormal conditions for a pregnant woman; shock; burns; fractures; and changes in level of consciousness.

Patient Flow

Patient flow refers to the management of the process and time required for the patient's agency visit from check-in in the reception area, to the time spent in the clinical examination area, to check-out. Efficient patient flow is associated with favorable patient satisfaction and enhanced agency revenues.

- Patient needs and preferences: The patients' needs affect daily patient flow when additional patients are scheduled for emergent or urgent care, or when the time required for the care of an individual patient exceeds the allotted time frame for the visit.

  Patient preferences may affect patient flow by creating competition for appointments at times that are considered most convenient, i.e., at 10 A.M. as opposed to 7:00 A.M.

- Physician preferences: The physician's preferences for amount of time spent in clinical practice affect patient flow independently of the allotted time for specific patient needs. The physician's preferences for completing documentation also influence patient flow. Some providers complete all necessary documentation for a patient before proceeding to care for the next scheduled patient. Other providers leave the completion of extensive documentation until the end of the day. The CMA accommodates each of these approaches In the scheduling matrix.

- Facility and equipment requirements: All aspects of the patient experience, from the availability of adequate parking to the numbers of available support staff, affect patient flow in the primary care practice. Patient flow procedures must be designed to minimize congestion in the reception area by providing separate areas for patients who are checking in and out, and to minimize patient wait time in the reception area and in the examining rooms. The CMA may be responsible for maintaining and documenting time checks to measure patient flow times from one point of the patient encounter to the completion of the patient visit. Providers can use this data to measure agency efficiency and to revise and improve patient flow practices.

<u>Outside Services</u>

In most instances, the CMA schedules laboratory and imaging studies, and outpatient diagnostic procedures for the patient. Surgical procedures and hospital admissions are scheduled by the CMA. Large surgical practices often employ a CMA to function as a dedicated admission coordinator.

To schedule outpatient laboratory, imaging, and diagnostic procedures, the CMA collects the necessary information that includes: the patient's name, contact information, the procedure to be performed, the reason for the order, the requested time frame for completion of the test or procedure, informed consent documents, and insurance details related to any necessary written referrals or preauthorization. Once the appointment details are established the CMA must contact the patient to review and confirm the date, time, location, and directions for the testing. The CMA also reviews the instructions for any patient preparations that are required prior to the examination. The patient also should be provided with written instructions by mail or in person well in advance of the testing date. The CMA documents the details of this pre-procedure notification process in the EHR, as well as the details of the patient's notification of the testing results. The CMA recognizes that this documentation is an important protection against claims of malpractice or patient abandonment.

The CMA understands that the patient's medical record must contain all required data to validate the reason for hospital admission. This data includes all provider documentation, laboratory testing and imaging results, informed consent documents, prescription history, and any additional data that relates to the patient's admitting diagnosis. The CMA is also responsible for obtaining preauthorization from the insurer, and the CMA is aware that failure to verify insurance details prior to admission can result in the patient being responsible for all costs of care. Once the appropriate information has been collected, the CMA verifies all admission details with the hospital's admissions department. When the admission is for an elective procedure, the CMA attempts to honor the patient's requests for specific days; however, the hospital is ultimately responsible for the final schedule. Depending on the circumstances, the CMA faxes the admitting orders to the admissions department at the hospital or to the appropriate nursing unit. Once the admission schedule is confirmed, the CMA provides the patient with an information packet that includes the details for the patient's admission, including directions to the hospital, parking and patient registration instructions, requirements for pre-operative testing if ordered, visiting hours and regulations, and the date and time for a post-operative check-up visit with the provider. The CMA documents a list of the instructions and the method used to inform the patient of these instructions in the EHR.

Appointment Protocols

<u>Legal Aspects</u>

The CMA understands that the appointment book, in either paper or digital form, is a legal document that is discoverable by the IRS and insurance providers. The daily schedule must be printed in some legible format, posted in a secure position, and corrected as necessary in the prescribed manner. The daily schedule serves as a record of all patients that were seen by the providers, as well as all patients that canceled and rescheduled appointments, patients that canceled but did not reschedule appointments, and patients that were "no-shows." The CMA consults with agency providers periodically to review the list of patients that did not keep their scheduled appointments and the CMA contacts those patients as directed by the providers. All efforts to contact the patient are documented in the EHR.

Physician Referrals

The CMA schedules all patients referred to the agency as soon as possible, communicates directly with the new patient, confirms all insurance information, and verifies that all patient data is appropriately prepared for the provider's use prior to the patient's appointment. The CMA also forwards all resulting patient data to the referring physician as appropriate.

When an established patient is referred to another provider, the CMA gathers all relevant documentation, confers with the responsible person in the provider's agency, and schedules the patient's appointment. When possible, the patient's preference for date and time for the appointment is accommodated. If necessary, the CMA provides a written referral for the patient's appointment. The CMA provides the patient with the details for the appointment in person or in written form as appropriate. The details should include location, directions, contact numbers, and any additional pre-visit requirements.

Cancelations and No-Shows

The CMA keeps a daily record of the patients that cancel and reschedule an appointment, patients that cancel an appointment without rescheduling the appointment, and patients that are "no-shows." The provider establishes an agency protocol to address the contact methods for patients that do not comply with recommended follow-up appointments, or patients who are consistent no-shows for scheduled appointments. The CMA understands that all attempts to contact these patients must be documented in the EHR to avoid possible charges of patient abandonment or malpractice. If the provider decides to dismiss the patient from the agency, the CMA sends the provider letter by certified mail and includes the signed receipt in the patient's EHR.

Physician Delay or Unavailability

If the physician becomes unavailable, the CMA reschedules all patients as soon as possible. If a provider is delayed, the CMA confers with patients present in the reception area to advise them of the delay and to reschedule the appointments per the patients' preferences. The CMA anticipates the patients' concerns related to the inconvenience and makes every effort to accommodate their requests.

Reminders or Recall Systems

Reminders or recall systems are designed to reduce the incidence of "no-shows" and to facilitate patient flow by ensuring the timely arrival of all patients. The CMA makes phone calls, provides written reminders to patients at check-out, and verifies that all appointment information is posted on patient portals. Agency providers must periodically assess the effectiveness of these various methods.

The CMA also uses the computerized EHR system to identify and schedule patients for routine examinations.

- Appointment cards: A printed card for future appointments should be given to patients when they check out. Depending on the intervening time frame and the patient's preference, the CMA sends a reminder card by mail to the patient two weeks prior to the next appointment.

- Phone calls, text messages, and e-mail notifications: The CMA makes phone calls or sends text and e-mail reminders depending on patient preferences and the pre-appointment interval designated by the agency. The e-mail messages may take the form of patient portal notifications which eliminates the need for individual providers to maintain current e-mail contact information for all patients. The CMA identifies and records patient preferences related to the messaging.

- Tickler file: The CMA maintains a chronologically oriented reminder or tickler file to facilitate the completion of repetitive tasks. Routine maintenance schedules for office equipment, employee certification schedules, and regulatory data submission schedules may be included in a tickler file.

Finances

Financial Terminology

Accounts Receivable
Accounts receivable is money owed to the agency by its debtors, e.g., insurance companies and patients.

Accounts Payable
Accounts payable are monies owed to vendors and may be designated as current liabilities. Accounts payable do not include contractual liabilities such as salaries.

Assets
Assets are goods, possessions, or property that have value. Primary care practice assets may include real estate, medical equipment, furnishings, and office equipment.

Liabilities
Liabilities are monies owed by the primary care practice.

Aging of Accounts
The list of accounts receivable aging identifies the unpaid invoices by for a certain time period. Any overdue payments are identified by this time-sensitive report.

Debit
As an accounting procedure, a debit either increases an asset or decreases a liability.

Credits
As an accounting procedure, a credit either decreases an asset or increases a liability.

Diagnosis Related Groups (DRGs)
DRGs include more than 500 possible diagnoses related to 20 body systems that are used as the basis of a statistical model for hospital reimbursement by Medicare. Payment is made per the DRG classification rather than the actual cost of care.

Relative Value Units (RVUs)
The RVUs are the end result of the calculations included in the Resource-based Relative Value Scale. RVUs are a measure of Medicare reimbursement relative to the value of physicians' services according to the current procedural terminology (CPT) for each service provided or each episode of care. The Centers for Medicaid and Medicare Services (CMS) annually evaluates three phases of medical services and procedures provided by physicians: physician work, practice expense, and malpractice expense. Each of these three elements is assigned a value that is designated as an RVU. Each of the RVUs is multiplied by the geographic cost practices indices (GCPI), which adjusts the reimbursement schedule

for geographic differences in the costs of providing care in more expensive areas of the country. In the final calculation, each of the three numbers is multiplied by the annually adjusted CMS physician fee schedule conversion factor, which was set at $35.89 in 2017.

Financial Procedures

Payment Receipts
- Co-pays: The co-pay is the amount of money that the patient must pay at each visit. The patient is responsible for understanding the terms of the third-party payer plan; however, the CMA should also be familiar with the requirements of plans that are common to the agency, to decrease errors in the collection of co-pays. In general, higher insurance premiums are associated with lower patient co-pays. The CMA collects and documents the receipt of all co-pays and secures the cash per agency policy.

Data Entry
- Post charges: The CMA understands that accurate posting of patient charges requires knowledge of the terms of the patient's insurance coverage, complete documentation of all care rendered by the agency providers, correct medical coding of all procedures, and knowledge of the agency fees for service. All these elements must be accurate and complete to prevent denial of the insurance claim for the visit.

- Post payments: The CMA examines all payment statements to confirm that all procedures that were initially billed were reimbursed at the correct rate. In addition, the CMA identifies any denied claims and reviews the explanatory information. Once the charges and the payment data have been reconciled, the CMA identifies any outstanding patient charges and processes those invoices, which must contain details of all procedures provided, incurred charges, and insurance adjustments.

- Post adjustments: The CMA understands that the adjusted collection rate is equal to the total reimbursement received from an insurer based on the agency's contractual agreement as compared to the total amount that should have been collected if there were no lost revenue issues inherent in the agency billing cycle.

Manage Petty Cash Account
Providers establish the rules for the petty cash account; however, the CMA understands that limiting the accessibility of the cash to a small number of staff members decreases the opportunity for mishandling of the funds. All additions and withdrawals should be witnessed by two people, with bank receipts attached to a permanent log book or file. Many agencies only accept credit or debit card payments for patient co-pays, which eliminates many of the management issues associated with the petty cash account.

Financial Calculations
The CMA may be responsible for calculating agency financial statements if they are educationally prepared to do so.

Billing Procedures
- Itemized statements: The CMA verifies that all billing statements issued in the name of the agency contain documentation of all procedures and costs, any insurance adjustments, and instructions for addressing any questions or concerns related to the charges.

- Billing cycle: The CMA understands that the key elements of the billing cycle include the processes related to patient check-in, verification of insurance coverage, accurate coding of the patient's diagnosis and procedures, calculation and entry of charges, claims submission, and posting of the payment. The CMA also understands that a documentation error or omission at any point in the cycle adversely affects the entire process.

Collection Procedures
- Aging of accounts: The CMA uses the accounts receivable aging report to identify the outstanding balances owed to the agency by insurance companies, patients, or other entities. The report lists the balances based on elapsed time since the billing date or due date, and the CMA understands that there is a correlation between the number of entries on the aging report and the financial vitality of the agency.

- Preplanned payment options: The CMA recognizes that the average patient with insurance coverage still may incur large out-of-pocket expenses because deductibles, co-payments, and costs not covered by the policy have increased dramatically. Agencies that do not collect the monies owed by the patient "up front" risk the development of bad debt that requires the use of a collection agency, which potentially harms the reputation of the provider and the agency. Providers must communicate effectively with all patients to identify actual costs and establish an equitable payment plan. The CMA understands that some of these options include; no-interest financing, payment discounts for up-front payments, and on-line payment options. The CMA provides information and empathetic financial counseling to identify the best solution for every patient.

- Credit arrangements: The provider develops a payment option for patient fees to decrease the occurrence of bad debts. The CMA implements these policies, which typically allow the patient to pay a portion of the total fee each month. This income decreases the patient's total interest charges and contributes a steady flow of income for the agency.

- Use of collection agencies: The CMA understands that while the services of a collection agency may be necessary at times, satisfying the debt by offering the patient alternative payment options often leads to a more favorable outcome.

Diagnostic and Procedural Coding Applications

Current Procedural Terminology (CPT)
CPT is a standardized coding scheme that facilitates the reporting of medical, surgical, and diagnostic procedures for payment.

- Modifiers: The CMA understands that a CPT modifier refines the original CPT definition of the procedure to reflect some addition or alteration in the original category. Modifiers add details to the original CPT that more closely reflect the patient encounter, which increases revenue and decreases the potential for denial of services.

- Upcoding: The CMA recognizes that upcoding refers to the fraudulent practice of reporting a CPT that represents a higher level of care or more complex diagnosis than is supported by the patient's diagnosis or EHR and provider documentation. The level of service for evaluation and management of a single patient encounter is coded according to the complexity of the care. The CMA understands that an example of upcoding could be using a level 5 code to report the care of a patient with a minor complaint for a brief encounter.

- Bundling of charges: Bundling of charges or episode-based payments is a reimbursement plan that reimburses providers for all episodes of care for an individual disease, diagnosis, or condition. For instance, the provider receives one payment for all outpatient and inpatient care for the patient with a total knee replacement, which contrasts with the traditional fee-for-service plan that includes charges and reimbursement for each care encounter or procedure. Proponents of the episode-based payment model view it as a cost savings measure that can contribute to improved patient outcomes, and positive provider and patient satisfaction. The potential cost savings are based on three assumptions: the contracted cost for episode-based care is less than fee-for-service cost for the same care; the savings that are generated are divided between the provider and the payer; and complications associated with the compensated illness or condition are not reimbursed. In addition, when hospitals participate in the episode-based payment model, providers who do not contract for bundled payment options that care for patients during a hospital stay receive fees for that care from the hospital, not the third-party payer.

International Classification of Diseases, Clinical Modifications (ICD-CM)

The international Classification of Diseases was developed by the World Health Organization (WHO) to provide a standardized coding system used to describe illnesses and conditions to be used worldwide to improve documentation, track epidemiological health trends and facilitate reimbursement strategies. In the United States, the coding system is divided into two separate systems that address hospital care (ICD-CM) and outpatient care (ICD-PCS). The ICD-9 system was revised and the ICD-10 system was endorsed by the membership of the World Health Organization in 1990; however, implementation in the United States has been delayed several times by congressional action due to the burden of the implementation of the revisions.

The ICD-9 included 18,000 disease and condition codes, while the ICD-10 contains 155,000 different codes. This increase is due to the specificity of the revised system. For instance, in ICD-9 there was a code for a fractured arm; in ICD-10 there is a code for a fractured right arm and a code for a fractured left arm. There are codes to identify subtle descriptors of all diseases and conditions, which has increased not only the number of codes, but also the complexity of the code itself. Formerly, ICD-9 codes were some combination of three- to five-digit alphanumeric characters, while ICD-10 codes are three- to seven-digit alphanumeric characters. Although providers and agencies completed implementation of the ICD-10 codes in 2015, more than thirty years after the original endorsement of the revisions, the World Health Organization is set to begin revision of the ICD-10 in 2017.

Linking Procedure and Diagnosis Codes

The CMA must maintain expertise in coding procedures, with attention to any agency specific coding requirements and contracted inclusions for the evidence-based care model. The coded entries must be justified by, and consistent with the patient's diagnosis as documented in the EHR. In addition, the CMA verifies that all appropriate codes are applied to each individual patient encounter for accurate reimbursement.

Healthcare Common Procedure Coding System

The Healthcare Common Procedure Coding System (HCPCS) is an additional standardized coding system used to provide a reimbursement framework for goods and services billed to Medicare and Medicaid and other third-party payers that are not included in the CPT codes issued by the American Medical Association) and are used outside the physician's office. These items may include ambulance charges, durable medical equipment such as prosthetics and orthotics, and associated supplies.

Third-Party Payers and Insurance

A third-party payer is any public or private organization that provides health insurance coverage for an individual patient. The providers negotiate contract terms with the payers for services, and the patients pay premiums to the payers in exchange for care by the provider. The contracts between individual agencies and third-party payers are subject to state and federal statutes. In addition, the CMA recognizes that the relationship between the agency and the third-party payers is also influenced by demands of the healthcare market, where providers require adequate compensation for the care provided and third-party payers are focused on managing costs. The CMA understands that the contracts that are negotiated with third-party payers are affected many diverse factors which may include: the amount of risk the providers are willing to assume in the form of episode-based care or other reimbursement models, the size of the agency and the clinical specialty services provided by that agency (which may mean that payers "need" the agency to enter the market in that location), and the agency's patient outcomes standards. The CMA knows that successful negotiation, accurate coding, and thorough documentation are all required for cost-effective practice.

Types of Plans

- Commercial plans: The CMA is aware that there are multiple variations and coverage criteria for third-party payer plans; however, most plans take the form of a health maintenance organization (HMO) or a preferred provider organization (PPO). An HMO assumes all financial risk and provides all care for its members in return for a fixed, pre-paid fee. An individual HMO is most often located in a specific geographic location. Variations of the HMO structure and function include group, staff, or network models. The group model includes salaried physicians from a single specialty group that provides patient care at per capita negotiated rates. In the staff model, the patient has access to a limited number of physicians who are employees of the HMO, and all care is provided in HMO-owned facilities. In the network model the HMO contracts with several physician groups to provide care for its members. The physicians in the contracted groups may provide care for HMO members as well as non-members.

  In the PPO model, patients receive care from a network of selected physicians who contract for that care with the third-party payer. Patients may access care from providers outside of the network, but most often there are increased deductibles and co-payments, and additional non-discounted charges for that care.

- Government plans: Health care insurance plans that are administered by individual state governments and the federal government include Medicare and Medicaid.

  - Medicare: Medicare covers all individuals over the age of sixty-five and all patients with end-stage renal disease. It also provides hospital insurance coverage and additional medical insurance coverage. Most patients who are eligible for Part A and Part B Medicare opt to enroll in Medicare Advantage plans that offer all covered Medicare services in addition to optional coverage for medications and other services. The organizational structure and financial stability of third-party payers that offer these supplementary plans must be initially reviewed and approved by Medicare. The Medicare Advantage plans are often hybrid models of the HMO and PPO care models.

- Advanced beneficiary notice: Advanced beneficiary notices (ABNs) of non-coverage of rendered care by Medicare apply only to individuals with original Medicare coverage. All patients enrolled in the Medicare Advantage plans receive a notice of Medicare non-coverage in the event that the provider does not believe that Medicare will allow the claim. The CMA must generate an ABN whenever the medical necessity requirements for the care or procedure are not met. That means that every procedure or service must be supported by documentation of the required clinical manifestation or patient complaint to meet the necessary and reasonable standard for that care. ABNs are not generated for procedures that are never covered by Medicare. The CMA must provide the patient with an ABN when the standard is not met, and the CMA documents the notification process in the EHR.

- Providers may voluntarily issue an ABN, and the CMA is aware that patients' preferences often result in denied claims at one of three points in the care relationship. The three points are initiation, reduction, and termination. For example, at the beginning of a care relationship a patient may request a prescription for physical therapy that is not supported by the provider's documentation, or once a therapy is ordered and the frequency of treatments is eventually decreased or the therapy is terminated, the patient may request that the that the therapy be continued even though the request no longer meets the necessary and reasonable standard.

- Medicaid: Medicaid is a federally mandated plan that is administered by individual states, which means that the CMA must be familiar with applicable state laws for these programs. Medicaid plans cover low-income individuals and certain protected populations. Depending on the details of the negotiated contracts with an individual state, the plan may resemble a fee-for-service plan or an HMO. Many more individuals became eligible for Medicaid as a result of the Affordable Care Act (ACA); however, the temporary provider reimbursement increases have expired and fewer providers are willing to care for patients covered by Medicaid.

- Tricare: Tricare is a federally administered insurance program for service members, reservists, dependents, and some retirees. The options for coverage are similar to other commercial plans with respect to networks, deductibles, and co-pays. There are also optional plans for dental coverage for active and reservist members.

- Civil Health and Medical Program of the Department of Veterans Affairs (CHAMPVA) covers dependents of veterans who are 100% permanently disabled as a result of their active duty, or dependents of veterans who have died as a result of a disability that resulted from active duty.

- Managed care organizations (MCOs): MCOs are medical insurers that negotiate contracts with providers and healthcare agencies to provide cost-effective care for plan members. All members understand that the MCO sets deductibles, co-payments, referral procedures, and access to the network of providers. In addition, members when members receive care outside of the MCO network, they incur additional expense. In general, the more flexible plans are associated with increased premiums. MCOs exist in three forms: HMOs, PPOs, and point of service plans (POS plans) that allow members to choose either the HMO or PPO option each time they access care. Most HMO plans reimburse in-network care only, while PPO plans reimburse in-network care at a higher rate than out-of-network care.

- Managed care requirements: The CMA recognizes that the individual MCOs have varied requirements for the plan members and the providers. Although the patients are ultimately responsible for understanding the terms of their contract with the MCO, the CMA can minimize the incidence of denied claims by maintaining current with the MCO requirements for the payers that contract with the agency.

  The contract between the MCO and the provider defines covered expenses, the definition of medical necessity, the grievance or appeals process for denied claims, requirements for preauthorization or pre-certification for treatment, and the definition of the standard of care. Providers require explicit information for each of these issues. As a first step in the contract negotiation process, providers must identify the financial status, ownership, community and patient reputation, and accreditation status of the MCO. The provider also must review all enrollment procedures for the MCO including printed media that explains plan options. The MCO should provide clear instructions for appeals of denied claims and the process of de-enrolling patients from the plan. The standard of care and the concept of medical necessity as it relates to covered expenses are critical issues that providers must consider in the process of contract negotiation. If a provider determines that a procedure or test is medically necessary even though it is not a covered expense under the contract, the provider's agency then assumes all the financial risks to meet that standard of care. Providers must also contract to provide only the care that can be reasonably provided with existing resources, including provider expertise, staffing quotas, and facilities.

  - Care referrals: All HMOs and many other MCOs require providers to consult with the MCO before ordering outpatient procedures such as physical therapy or referring the patient to a specialty provider. After the MCO has been notified, the patient may obtain a referral for the treatment or visit. The CMA understands that while most MCOs allow phone messaging for the referral process, the process is specific to the individual MCO contract, and the CMA verifies that all patient referrals comply with the individual MCO.

  - Pre-certification: Pre-certification is the process of demonstrating the medical necessity of a patient's admission to an acute care facility. The provider is responsible for documentation that supports the need for admission, and for contacting the MCO to verify the details of the patient's condition. The CMA is responsible for verifying that all required documentation is complete, accurate, and forwarded to the appropriate hospital representative and to the MCO as necessary. The CMA also communicates the details of the admission and any additional information to the patient and the patient's family.

    Pre-certification is also required for various diagnostic tests such as CT scans, MRIs, or PET scans, and outpatient surgical procedures such as cataract surgery and cochlear implants. The CMA recognizes and satisfies the pre-certification requirements for the individual MCOs.

- Prior authorization: To contain costs, prevent drug interactions, and provide patients with the best therapy, MCOs also require prior authorization for prescription medications under certain conditions. The provider must obtain prior authorization for any medication that can be replaced by a generic drug with the same efficacy, for medications prescribed at higher than usual dosages, for medications that treat non-life threatening conditions, or for very expensive medications. The CMA makes every effort to process the preauthorization requests and any subsequent appeals for coverage in a timely manner to ensure that patients receive the prescribed medications.

- Workers' compensation: Workers' compensation insurance reimburses providers for the care of individuals with injuries related to their employment. A claims adjuster who represents the workers' compensation commercial carrier is assigned to the patient when a claim is made. The adjuster will initially determine whether the patient is cared for by their primary care physician or by a provider representing the workers' compensation carrier. The adjuster then is responsible for authorizing all care requests from the provider. The CMA understands that the procedure for filing workers' compensation claims is state mandated and that the claims are completed as pen and paper documents that are mailed to the carrier rather than submitted electronically. Timely agency reimbursement for care of an individual whose care is covered by workers' compensation requires accurate and comprehensive documentation of all care and proper submission of complete, accurate, and legible handwritten forms. Only the carrier of the workers' compensation insurance is billed for care that is provided for the work-related injury. The patient's private insurer is billed for services not associated with that injury that are provided while the patient is receiving the pre-authorized care.

Insurance Claims
- Submission: The CMA understands that the submission of a claim to a third-party payer is an intricate process that relies on comprehensive documentation in the EHR, identification of all applicable ICD-10 and CPT codes, accurate preparation of all accompanying documentation required by the individual insurer, and timely electronic submission of the completed claim. Errors or omissions in any step of the process can result in denial of the claim, which interrupts the agency revenue cycle.

- Appeals and denials: The first time that MCOs deny a claim, the decision is based on whether the claim is within the plan guidelines. Providers should recognize that the most common reason for denial is improper documentation. Providers are encouraged to communicate directly with the reviewer to explain extenuating circumstances and to include a summary letter that clearly defines the details of the claim. If the appeal is rejected, the provider understands that a second appeal is reviewed independently of the details of the insurance plan. This means that the provider who references peer-reviewed evidence in the summary letter to support the original treatment or service is more likely to achieve a favorable decision. Patient participation in the appeals process is discouraged because, in the first appeal, reviewers are only comparing the provider's documentation to the details of the plan, and the patient is not able to contribute any substantive information to that inquiry. The CMA understands that the most important part of the claims process is the accuracy of the documentation that supports the coding.

- Explanation of benefits (EOB): The CMA understands that MCOs issue periodic statements to patients that include claims and reimbursement details for care provided for a specific time period. Insurers view this document as protection against fraud and abuse because the patient can identify procedures or services that were provided. Many MCOs provide forms that include all billing codes; however, the CMS distributes a Medicare Summary Notice every three months to all Medicare recipients that uses simple language to identify the claims.

Practice Questions

1. What is one of the main differences between the POMR and the SOMR?
    a. Only nurses can add data to the SOMR.
    b. The POMR facilitates the assessment of patient outcomes.
    c. The SOMR generates less paper.
    d. The POMR separates the notes from each discipline.

2. Which of the following statements best identifies the meaningful use initiative?
    a. The plan provides financial rewards to providers for better patient outcomes.
    b. The initiative is focused on decreasing medication errors.
    c. The meaningful use initiative requires the use of the SOMR for compliance.
    d. The development and use of the electronic health record is the focus of the initiative.

3. Which of the following elements is NOT required to schedule an appointment for an established patient?
    a. The patient's height and weight
    b. The patient's current complaint
    c. The provider's vacation schedule
    d. The dates of national holidays

4. The problem list generated in a POMR is most often displayed as a database. Which of the categories is an essential element of that database?
    a. The patient's age
    b. The date of onset of the problem
    c. The list of the patient's previous medications
    d. The patient's weight

5. Which of the following is an appropriate order of events for a CMA to do with a patient whose provider has decided to dismiss the patient from the agency?
    a. The CMA should send the patient a letter by certified mail and include the patient's "no-show" schedule with the provider's list of specific complaints.
    b. The CMA should find the patient in person and tell them face-to-face that the provider no longer wishes to see them.
    c. The CMA should send the patient a letter by certified mail and include the signed receipt of the patient's EHR.
    d. The CMA should email the patient their medical history and the detailed reason why they are being dismissed from the agency.

6. Which of the following statements correctly defines the criteria for an established patient for insurance purposes?
    a. The patient saw the provider one time, 5 years ago.
    b. The provider consulted on the patient's care in the hospital last month.
    c. The patient was seen by one provider 2 years ago and has a current EHR.
    d. The patient is being scheduled for a visit by a referring provider.

7. Which of the following is the most critical element of the documentation that is required to arrange a hospital admission?

   a. The patient's preference for the admission date
   b. The referring physician's specialty
   c. The patient's age
   d. EHR data that supports the need for admission

8. Which statement regarding "no-shows" is correct?

   a. People who consistently miss appointments may be dismissed from the primary care practice.
   b. The provider is legally required to report "no-shows" to the patient's insurance company.
   c. "No-shows" are not contacted about rescheduling.
   d. The provider may report the "no-show" to the insurance company, but only at the provider's discretion.

9. Which of the following statements best describes upcoding?

   a. Upcoding is a method that is used to upgrade the EHR to reflect the patient's current status.
   b. Upcoding is a coding modifier that indicates that more than one test was completed during the patient encounter.
   c. Upcoding is a coding method that reports a level of care that is not documented in the EHR.
   d. Upcoding is the process of updating CPT modifiers.

10. Which of the following correctly identifies individuals that are eligible for CHAMPVA insurance coverage?

    a. Dependents of active duty service members.
    b. Adult children of active duty service members.
    c. All retired veterans are eligible.
    d. Dependents of veterans who are 100% disabled due to their active duty.

11. Which of the following statements regarding the advanced beneficiary notice (ABN) is correct?

    a. The CMA sends the ABN to all Medicare recipients when preauthorization for a procedure is denied.
    b. ABNs are only sent to patients enrolled in original Medicare programs, not Medicare Advantage programs.
    c. A patient's request for therapy that does not meet the necessary and reasonable standard always requires an ABN.
    d. ABNs are only sent to patients for denied hospital claims.

12. Which of the following statements regarding preauthorization is correct?

    a. The requirement is waived for outpatient surgery.
    b. The provider assumes all financial risk if a service is provided without preauthorization.
    c. The provider must obtain preauthorization for all hospital admissions.
    d. Preauthorization is only required for Medicare patients.

13. Which of the following statements is one of the assumptions of the savings potential of the bundled payment model of reimbursement?

    a. Patient outcomes will not be affected by the bundled payment plan.
    b. The providers and payers will share the savings that result from the model.
    c. Patients will consume less health care.
    d. The providers will be reimbursed for complications of care.

14. Which of the following statements related to workers' compensation claims is correct?
    a. The CMA bills all the patient's care to the patient's private insurer first.
    b. The patient receives all care from their primary care provider.
    c. The CMA verifies that preauthorization for all care and procedures is obtained.
    d. All documentation will be electronically transmitted to the insurance carrier for the workers' compensation plan in the individual state.

15. Which of the following statements about Medicaid is correct?
    a. The federal government funds and sets the policies for the plan.
    b. The purpose of the plan is provide health care services for low-income individuals and families.
    c. All primary care providers are required to accept Medicaid patients.
    d. The Affordable Healthcare Act resulted in fewer people seeking Medicaid coverage.

16. Which of the following statements about HMO models is correct?
    a. The staff model and the group model have the same provider reimbursement structure.
    b. In the network model, patients receive care in HMO-owned medical facilities.
    c. Physicians in the network model provide care exclusively for HMO members.
    d. HMOs commonly exist in a single geographic area.

17. A patient asks the CMA to explain the use of Fluticasone with Salmeterol, the new medication that the provider just ordered. Which of the following responses is most appropriate?
    a. "Open the container, click the dose into position, take a deep breath, exhale, inhale the medication through the mouth, and hold your breath for 10 seconds."
    b. "It is best if you swallow the medication with a full glass of water."
    c. "Press the inhaler as you breathe in slowly, and then hold your breath for 10 seconds."
    d. "Be sure to take this medication with food to avoid nausea."

18. The medical identifies the agency responsibilities for blood-borne pathogen management. Which of the following statements is incorrect?
    a. "The Occupational Safety and Health Administration (OSHA) requires agencies to maintain employee training records."
    b. "All employees must be provided with appropriate personal protective equipment."
    c. "The agency must enforce universal precautions."
    d. "To facilitate a prompt response to any occupational exposure to a blood-borne pathogen, the agency will annually review and maintain all employees' medical records."

19. Which of the following correctly pairs the medication name with its description?
    a. Diclofenac, opioid analgesic
    b. Paroxetine, serotonin reuptake inhibitor (SSRI)
    c. Hydroxyzine, potassium-sparing diuretic
    d. Ondansetron, proton pump inhibitor

20. The CMA is admitting a 35-year-old male patient with a leg injury. The x-ray indicates that the tibia is fractured, and there is an open wound at the site of the fracture. Which of the following correctly identifies this injury?
    a. Compound
    b. Comminuted
    c. Stable
    d. Greenstick

21. The CMA is preparing to assist with a sterile procedure. After the outer packaging containing the sterile gloves is removed, what is the next step?

    a. Position the thumb against the palm of the hand and slip the hand into the glove.

    b. Position the fingers under the cuff of the glove and insert the hand.

    c. Pick up the inside cuff of the glove with the non-dominant hand.

    d. Open the inside sterile wrapper using the paper tabs.

22. The CMA receives a call from a patient stating that a child may have ingested an unknown cleaning agent. Which of the following is the CMA's best response?

    a. "Take the child to the hospital immediately."

    b. "Call the poison control center and follow their directions."

    c. "Try to induce vomiting with Ipecac."

    d." The doctor can see you right away."

23. The patient tells the CMA, "I don't understand how to take this new pill, the nitroglycerin, that my doctor just ordered." Which of the following is the CMA's best response?

    a. "Be sure to take the pill with food."

    b. "Grapefruit juice will interfere with the absorption of the pill."

    c. "The pill should be placed under your tongue and allowed to dissolve."

    d. "You should drink eight ounces of water with this pill to be sure it reaches the stomach."

24. The CMA works in a college health center. Providers in this setting must be alert for students exhibiting manifestations of meningitis. Which of the following symptoms are associated with this condition?

    a. Nuchal rigidity with headache

    b. Numbness and tingling in the hands and feet

    c. Right lower quadrant pain

    d. Hyperactivity

25. The CMA is assisting with the care of a patient with suspected myocardial infarction. The CMA correctly places the patient in which of the following anatomical positions?

    a. Lithotomy

    b. Trendelenburg

    c. Supine

    d. Semi-fowler's

Answer Explanations

1. B: The problem list in the POMR demonstrates the effect of the interventions on the resolution of the individual problems. This chronological record can be used as an outcome measure that is an essential element of the meaningful use standard. The SOMR does not specifically track the resolution of individual problems and therefore is less useful for outcomes assessment than the POMR. Any provider that renders care for the patient documents that care in the SOMR; therefore, Choice A is incorrect. There is no evidence that the SOMR generates less paper. In fact, the opposite may be true because each provider maintains a separate entry in the medical record; therefore, Choice C is incorrect. The POMR is a chronological compilation of the patient care documentation by all disciplines; therefore, Choice D is incorrect.

2. D: The meaningful use initiative is a government-funded incentive program that requires the development and implementation of the EHR. It is based on the assumption that the use of the EHR will positively impact the quality of patient care. The meaningful use initiative rewards are determined by the implementation of the EHR, rather than by patient outcomes. The CMA should be aware that there are other government-funded programs that reward providers for improved outcomes, and that it is why medical record models that facilitate outcomes assessment are commonly used by providers. However, Choice A is incorrect. The implementation of the EHR may improve patient care error rates; however that is not the basis for the meaningful use initiative; therefore, Choice B is incorrect. The meaningful use plan does not require a specific medical record model, but the literature seems to suggest that the POMR is superior to the SOMR regarding outcomes measurement; therefore, Choice C is incorrect.

3. A: The CMA should identify the patient's reason for requesting the appointment, consult the appointment matrix to be sure that the provider is available, and determine whether the agency is open on the intended date. The patient's height and weight are not required for scheduling an appointment.

4. B: The database entries should include the problem, the date of onset, the interventions, and the date of resolution of the problem. The problem list is a chronological record of the patient's progress from the time of the current interventions, which means that details such as the patient's weight and previous medications have already been considered in the development of the problem list. Therefore, Choices A, C, and D are incorrect.

5. C: The CMA should send the patient a letter by certified mail and include the signed receipt of the patient's EHR. The CMA should not find the patient face-to-face or send them a list with their provider's complaints, making Choices A and B incorrect. The information should be sent by mail, not email, making Choice D incorrect.

6. C: Insurance regulations define an established patient as an individual who has been seen by at least one provider in the previous three years and has an EHR generated by that agency. Choice A is therefore incorrect, because the previous encounter was more than 3 years ago. If a provider cares for the patient in the hospital, the documentation of that care would be included in the patient's hospital record; however, the patient would not have a current record within the agency. That means that if the patient were to schedule an agency appointment with the provider, the patient would be considered a new patient; therefore, Choice B is incorrect. A patient referred to a provider in the agency is considered a new patient, rather than an established patient; therefore, Choice D is incorrect.

7. D: All the data is included in the pre-admission documentation; however, if the EHR does not contain adequate data to support the medical necessity for the admission, the patient is responsible for all care costs. Therefore, Choice *D* is the highest priority among the four choices.

8. A: Patients who consistently miss appointments or cancel without rescheduling the appointment may be considered non-compliant with the health care plan and may be dismissed by the provider after proper notice is provided. Therefore Choice *A* is correct. The CMA attempts to reschedule all missed appointments, including those identified as "no-shows." The patient's attendance pattern is not reported to the insurer, so Choices *B* and *D* are incorrect. However, the provider may impose a fee for the missed appointments.

9. C: Upcoding is the fraudulent practice of reporting a level of care delivered in a patient encounter that is not supported by the EHR or the patient's diagnosis. Upcoding is discoverable in routine audits and the provider may be penalized. The EHR reflects the patient's status as a result of accurate documentation by all providers; therefore, Choice *A* is incorrect. Modifiers are standardized: two numerical or two alpha character symbols are used to refine the definition of the initial code. Therefore, Choice *B* is incorrect. The CPT modifiers are updated by the American Medical Association's CPT Editorial Panel; therefore, Choice *D* is incorrect.

10. D: CHAMPVA insurance coverage covers only the dependents of veterans who are 100% disabled as a result of their active duty, or the dependents of deceased veterans who were 100% disabled as a result of their active duty. Therefore, Choices *A*, *B*, and *C* are incorrect.

11. B: The ABN is the form that is sent to patients enrolled in original Medicare plans when a claim is denied by Medicare. Members of Medicare Advantage programs receive a Medicare Notice of Non-coverage when the CMA identifies the claim one that is likely to be denied. Therefore, Choice *A* is incorrect. A patient's request for therapy that does meet the necessary and reasonable status may be appealed and approved; therefore, Choice *C* is incorrect. Primary care providers only notify patients of primary care procedures that may be denied, not hospital procedures; therefore, Choice *D* is incorrect.

12. B: If a physician believes that a procedure or treatment is necessary but it is not a covered expense, the physician assumes financial responsibility for all costs associated with that treatment or procedure. Preauthorization is required for all treatments; pre-certification is required for hospital admission. Therefore Choices *A* and *C* are incorrect. Preauthorization applies to all patients insured by MCOs as stipulated by the individual plans; therefore, Choice *D* is incorrect.

13. B: The cost-saving potential for the bundled payment option is based on three assumptions: bundled payments will result in less expensive care, providers and payers will divide excess revenue generated by the plan, and providers will not be compensated for complications of covered conditions, which results in additional savings. Although not identified as the financial focus of the reimbursement plan, improved patient outcomes are also identified as possible favorable outcomes; therefore, Choice *A* is incorrect. The authors of the reimbursement plan expect that patients will receive more care and cost-effective care with improved patient outcomes; therefore, Choice *C* is incorrect. One of the basic assumptions of the cost-saving plan is that providers will not be reimbursed for complications of care; therefore Choice *D* is incorrect.

14. C: The CMA is responsible for obtaining preauthorization for all care and procedures. The CMA is also responsible for documentation that supports the necessary and reasonable standard in order to eliminate denials for care and reimbursement delays. The CMA understands that all covered expenses are billed to the workers' compensation commercial carrier. Services and care that are not directly associated with the patient's employment are submitted to the patient's third-party payer in accordance with that contract; therefore, Choice A is incorrect. The workers' compensation commercial carrier will assign a claims adjustor to all covered employees, and that adjustor will issue preauthorization for details of the patient's care, including the assignment of a primary care physician. That means that the patient may not see their own primary care physician; therefore, Choice B is incorrect. The CMA understands that the workers' compensation claim forms are completed as paper documents and are submitted directly to the commercial carrier; therefore, Choice D is incorrect.

15. B: Medicaid is intended to provide healthcare services for low-income individuals and families. The federal government funds the plan; however, the plan is administered by the individual states; therefore, Choice A is incorrect. Although a large number of providers do accept Medicaid reimbursement, physicians are not legally obligated to do so; therefore, Choice C is incorrect. The Affordable Healthcare Act revised the requirements for Medicaid eligibility, which resulted in a significant increase in the number of Medicaid recipients; therefore, Choice D is incorrect.

16. D: HMOs enroll members from a single geographic area, which may be localized to a city or a state. In the staff model, the physicians are employees of the HMO, and all patient care is provided in facilities owned by the HMO. In the group model, all physicians are salaried employees from a single specialty group that negotiates per capita care rates with the HMO; therefore, the reimbursement rates for the two models is not the same, so Choice A is incorrect. In the network group the HMO contracts with several physician groups to provide care for members. These providers care for non-member patients as well as member patients; therefore, Choice C is incorrect.

17. A: Fluticasone with Salmeterol (trade name: Advair Diskus) is an inhaled powder that is contained in a disk structure. The disk has a mouthpiece and a lever that positions the individual dose. The patient is instructed to inhale and exhale slowly before positioning the lips firmly around the mouthpiece. After the medication has been inhaled, the patient should hold their breath for ten seconds before slowly exhaling. The patient is instructed to rinse the mouth with water *without swallowing* after the medication is inhaled. Rinsing the medication from the oral cavity reduces the incidence of thrush, which may develop as a result of the residual medication in the mouth; therefore, Choice B is incorrect. Choice C identifies the procedure for using an inhaler that is used for medications other than Advair; therefore Choice C is incorrect. This medication is inhaled into the lungs, which means that food intake is not required; therefore Choice D is incorrect.

18. D: The agency does not review or maintain the medical records of the employees. In the event of an occupational exposure to HCV or HIV, and depending on applicable laws, the agency will test the blood of the source of the exposure and the exposed employee. The exposed worker will be offered appropriate prophylaxis for the causative agent, counseling, and ongoing assessment of any illnesses. The worker's healthcare provider will issue an opinion to the agency, and the worker's medical record will be kept in strict confidence. The remaining choices are OSHA requirements for all agencies; therefore Choices A, B, and C are incorrect.

19. B: Paroxetine is a psychotropic drug used to treat mood disorders such as depression and anxiety disorders. Diclofenac is a non-steroidal anti-inflammatory drug, rather than an opioid analgesic, which is used to treat mild to moderate pain such as the pain associated with osteoarthritis and rheumatoid arthritis; therefore Choice A is incorrect. Hydroxyzine is an antihistamine with antianxiety effects; therefore Choice C is incorrect. Ondansetron is an anti-emetic used for post-operative nausea and nausea associated with chemotherapy; therefore Choice D is incorrect.

20. A: A compound fracture is defined as a fractured bone that is associated with an open wound. The bone may or may not be visible in the wound. A comminuted fracture occurs when the bone is broken into three or more pieces; therefore, based on the information in the question, Choice *B* is incorrect. A stable fracture occurs when the proximal and distal ends of the fractured bone are not displaced, and there is no breakage in the skin; therefore Choice *C* is incorrect. Greenstick fractures are long bone fractures that are common in children less than 10 years of age. This fracture may be considered as an incomplete fracture because the soft bones bend; therefore Choice *D* is incorrect.

21. D: The correct sequence of steps for sterile gloving is:

1. Once the outer wrap is discarded, the sterile inner wrap is opened with the paper tabs.

2. The inner cuff of the glove is picked up by the non-dominant hand.

3. The thumb of the dominant hand is held flat against the palm.

4. The hand is slid into the glove.

5. The gloved hand slips under the cuff of the remaining glove.

6. The thumb is held against the palm and the hand is slid into the glove.

The question asks about the first step, what to do after removing the outer packaging. Choice *D* answers the question correctly; therefore, Choices *A*, *B*, and *C* are incorrect.

22. B: The only appropriate action is to instruct the mother to contact the poison control center. Transporting the child to the hospital or agency without any additional information about the poison can delay appropriate treatment; therefore Choices *A* and *D* are incorrect. Vomiting is contraindicated unless it is verified as a safe intervention for the identified poison; therefore Choice *C* is incorrect.

23. C: Nitroglycerin is formulated for sublingual (under the tongue) administration. The medication dissolves rapidly into the circulation and acts to dilate the coronary arteries in order to relieve the pain of angina. The remaining choices are not appropriate to the administration of nitroglycerin; therefore, Choices *A*, *B*, and *C* are incorrect.

24. A: The classic manifestation of meningitis is the nuchal rigidity (stiffness of the neck) that is associated with severe head pain. The head pain is due to the inflammation and irritation of the meninges by the causative organism. Skin rashes, fever, chills, nausea and vomiting, lethargy, and confusion are also associated with this infection. However, peripheral sensory changes, abdominal pain, and hyperactivity are not associated with meningitis; therefore Choices *B*, *C*, and *D* are incorrect.

25. D: Semi-fowler's is the position of choice to facilitate respiration in order to relieve chest pain by maximizing oxygen delivery to the heart. The lithotomy position is required for vaginal and pelvic examinations; therefore, Choice *A* is incorrect. Trendelenburg is the position for shock states when increased blood flow to the brain is required; therefore Choice *B* is incorrect. The supine position does not facilitate respiration and is not appropriate for the care of a patient with an MI; therefore Choice *C* is incorrect.

Clinical

Anatomy and Physiology

Body as a Whole

Animal cell

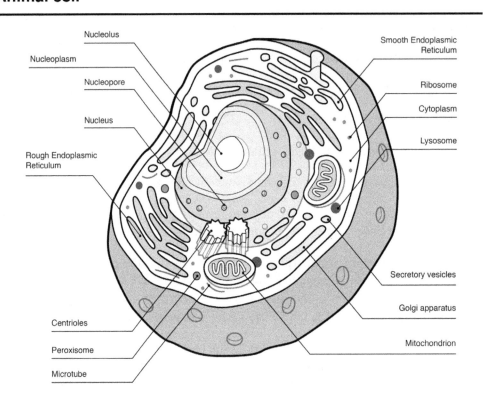

Nucleolus

Nucleoplasm

Nucleopore

Nucleus

Rough Endoplasmic
Reticulum

Centrioles

Peroxisome

Microtube

Smooth Endoplasmic
Reticulum

Ribosome

Cytoplasm

Lysosome

Secretory vesicles

Golgi apparatus

Mitochondrion

Structural Units

The structural units of the human body include the cells, tissues, organs, and organ systems. The **cell** is the basis for all life. The function of a specific cell type will dictate its structure; however, all cells have certain subunits or organelles in common. The nucleus directs all cellular activities and contains the DNA-specific chromosomes for the individual. The cell membrane provides a barrier between the cellular contents and the environment and regulates the substances that cross the membrane in either direction. The cytoplasm is the intracellular fluid where all cellular reactions occur. The mitochondria are responsible for energy production. The ribosomes create the proteins that are necessary for all bodily functions. The smooth endoplasmic reticulum creates lipids, which are necessary for cellular structure. The centrioles are responsible for cellular division and reproduction. The lysosomes synthesize and store digestive enzymes.

Tissues are groups of cells that perform specific functions. The four types of tissues are epithelial, muscle, connective, and nervous. Epithelial tissue covers the exterior surface of the body, lines the interior surfaces, and forms some glands. Muscle tissue is capable of movement as a result of electrical stimulation. There are three specialized types of muscle tissue: skeletal or voluntary muscle; smooth or involuntary muscle, found in hollow internal organs such as the bladder, lungs, and blood vessels; and cardiac muscle. Connective tissue connects all body systems and provides structural support. The skin, ligaments, and tendons are all composed of varying forms of connective tissue. Nervous tissue also responds to an electrical stimulus and can generate nerve impulses that result in voluntary and involuntary bodily functions.

An **organ** is a coordinated structure of various tissue types that performs a specific function for the body. An **organ system** is composed of two or more organs that contribute complementary functions to support the vital functions of the body. For example, the heart, lungs, and circulatory system work together to provide for oxygenation.

Anatomical Divisions, Body Cavities

Body Cavities	
Cavity	**Contents**
Dorsal Cavity (Posterior)	Brain
	Spinal Cord
Ventral (Anterior)	Includes the organs of the: Thoracic Cavity, Abdominal Cavity, and Pelvic Cavity
Thoracic Cavity	Heart, Lungs, and Thymus
Abdominal Cavity	Stomach, Liver, Gall Bladder, Spleen, Small Intestine, Kidneys, Large Intestine, Adrenal Gland
Pelvic Cavity	Urinary Bladder, Sigmoid Colon, Male and Female Reproductive Organs

Anatomical Positions and Directions
The basic anatomical position refers to the body standing straight, forward facing, with the upper extremities at the side and the palms forward facing. Specific body positions may be necessary to accommodate the patient's condition or planned interventions. In the **supine** position, the patient lies flat with straight knees and arms at the side. A variation of the supine position is the Fowler's position, which includes elevation of the head to approximately 30 to 45 degrees. In the **prone** position, the patient lays on the stomach with straight knees and the arms at the side or under the head. The dorsal recumbent and lithotomy positions are similar because in each position the patient lies flat with knees flexed and their feet either flat on the bed or resting in stirrups. The **knee-chest** and standing positions are also similar. The patient is bent at the waist, either standing or with knees resting on the bed. In the left-lateral or **Sim's** position, the patient lies on the left side with the right knee flexed. In the Trendelenburg position, the patient lies flat with the head lowered.

The anterior position indicates the front of the body. The posterior position is the opposite of anterior, meaning toward the back. Superior is toward the head, and inferior is toward the feet. Medial is closer to the midline of the body. Lateral is away from midline toward the side of the body. Proximal means closer to the center of the body. Distal means further from the center of the body. Superficial refers to the surface of the body. Deep is the opposite of superficial, meaning it is closer to the body core. Bilateral refers to two structures, with one on each side of the body. Ipsilateral means the same side of the body, and contralateral means the opposite side of the body.

Body Planes, Quadrants

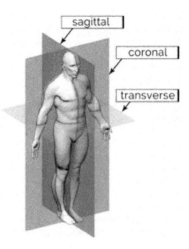

The coronal plane divides the body into the anterior, or frontal, and posterior, or dorsal, sections. The sagittal plane divides the body into left and right sections. The transverse plane divides the body into top and bottom sections.

For purposes of assessment, the abdomen is divided into four anatomical quadrants, as noted in the figure below to the right.

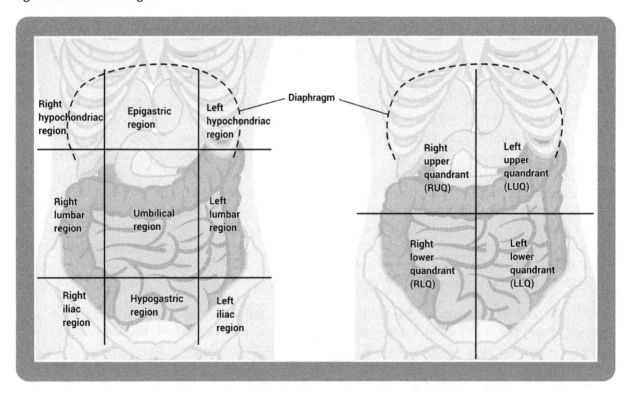

Body Systems and Their Normal Structure, Function, and Interrelationships Across the Life Span

Integumentary

The skin or integumentary body system is the largest organ of the body in surface area and weight. It is composed of three layers, which include the outermost layer or epidermis, the dermis, and the hypodermis. The thickness of the epidermis varies according to the specific body area. For example, the skin is thicker on the palms and the soles of the feet than on the eyelids. The dermis contains the hair follicles, sebaceous glands and sweat glands. Melanin is the pigment that is responsible for skin color.

The main function of the skin is the protection of the body from the outside environment. The skin regulates body temperature, using the insulation provided by body fat and the secretion of sweat, which acts as a coolant for the body. Sebum lubricates and protects the hair and the skin, and melanin absorbs harmful ultraviolet radiation. Special cells that lie on the surface of the skin also provide a barrier to bacterial infection. Nerves in the skin are responsible for sensations of pain, pressure, and temperature. In addition, the synthesis of Vitamin D, which is essential for the absorption of calcium from ingested food, begins in the skin.

Vernix caseosa is a thick, protein-based substance that protects the skin of the fetus against infection and irritation from the amniotic fluid from the third trimester until it dissipates after birth. Several childhood illnesses, such as measles and chicken pox, are associated with specific skin alterations. Acne related to hormonal changes is common in adolescents, and the effects of sunburn are observed across the life span. In the elderly, some of the protections provided by the skin become less effective; decreases in body fat and altered sweat production affect cold tolerance, loss of collagen support results in wrinkling of the skin, and decreased sebum secretions lead to changes in hair growth and skin moisture content.

Musculoskeletal
The musculoskeletal system consists of the bones, muscles, tendons, ligaments, and connective tissues that function together, providing support and motion of the body. The layers of bone include the hard exterior compact bone, the spongy bone that contains nerves and blood vessels, and the central bone marrow. The outer compact layer is covered by the strong periosteum membrane, which provides additional strength and protection for the bone. Skeletal muscles are voluntary muscles that are capable of contracting in response to nervous stimulation. Muscles are connected to bones by tendons, which are composed of tough connective tissue. Additional connective tissues called ligaments connect one bone to another at various joints.

In addition to providing support and protection, the bones are important for calcium storage and the production of blood cells. Skeletal muscles allow movement by pulling on the bones, while joints make different body movements possible.

The two most significant periods of bone growth are during fetal life and at puberty. However, until old age, bone is continually being remodeled. Specialized cells called osteoclasts break down the old bone, and osteoblasts generate new bone. In the elderly, bone remodeling is less effective, resulting in the loss of bone mass, and the incidence of osteoporosis increases. These changes can result in bone fractures, often from falling, that do not heal effectively. Muscle development follows a similar pattern with a progressive increase in muscle mass from infancy to adulthood, as well as a decline in muscle mass and physical strength in the elderly.

Nervous
The two parts of the nervous system are the central nervous system, which contains the brain and spinal cord, and the peripheral nervous system, which includes the ganglia and nerves. The cerebrospinal fluid and the bones of the cranium and the spine protect the brain and spinal cord. The nerves transmit impulses from one another to accomplish voluntary and involuntary processes. The nerves are

surrounded by a specialized myelin sheath that insulates the nerves and facilitates the transmission of impulses.

The nervous system receives information from the body, interprets that information, and directs all motor activity for the body. This means the nervous system coordinates all the activities of the body.

The fetal brain and spinal cord are clearly visible within six weeks after conception. After the child is born, the nervous system continues to mature as the child gains motor control and learns about the environment. In the well-elderly, brain function remains stable until the age of eighty, when the processing of information and short-term memory may slow.

Cardiovascular, Hematopoietic, and Lymphatic

The cardiovascular system includes the heart, the blood vessels, and the blood. The heart is a muscle that has four "chambers," or sections. The three types of blood vessels are: the arteries, which have a smooth muscle layer and are controlled by the nervous system; the veins, which are thinner than arteries and have valves to facilitate the return of the blood to the heart; and the capillaries, which are often only one-cell thick. Blood is red in color because the red blood cells (RBCs) that carry oxygen contain hemoglobin, which is a red pigment.

The deoxygenated blood from the body enters the heart and is transported to the lungs to allow the exchange of waste products for oxygen. The oxygenated blood then returns to the heart, which pumps the blood to the rest of body. The arteries carry oxygenated blood from the heart to the body; the veins return the deoxygenated blood to the heart, while the actual exchange of oxygen and waste products takes place in the capillaries.

The fetal cardiac system must undergo dramatic changes at birth as the infant's lungs function for the first time. Cardiovascular function remains stable until middle age, when genetic influences and lifestyle choices may affect the cardiovascular system. Most elderly people have at least some indication of decreasing efficiency of the system.

The hematopoietic system, a division of the lymphatic system, is responsible for blood-cell production. The cells are produced in the bone marrow, which is soft connective tissue in the center of large bones that have a rich blood supply. The two types of bone marrow are red bone marrow and yellow bone marrow.

The red bone marrow contains the stem cells, which can transform into specific blood cells as needed by the body. The yellow bone marrow is less active and is composed of fat cells; however, if needed, the yellow marrow can function as the red marrow to produce the blood cells.

The red bone marrow predominates from birth until adolescence. From that point on, the amount of red marrow decreases, and the amount of yellow marrow increases. This means that the elderly are at risk for conditions related to decreased blood-cell replenishment.

The lymphatic system includes the spleen, thymus, tonsils, lymph nodes, lymphatic vessels, and the lymph. The spleen is located below the diaphragm and to the rear of the stomach. The thymus consists of specialized lymphatic tissue and lies in the mediastinum behind the sternum. The tonsils are globules of lymphoid tissue located in the oropharynx. The lymphatic vessels are very small and contain valves to prevent backflow in the system vessels. The vessels that lie in close proximity to the capillaries circulate the lymph. Lymph is composed of infectious substances and cellular waste products in addition to hormones and oxygen.

The main function of the lymphatic system is protection against infection. The system also conserves body fluids and proteins and absorbs vitamins from the digestive system.

The spleen filters the blood in order to remove toxic agents and is also a reservoir for blood that can be released into systemic circulation as needed. The thymus is the site of the development and regulation of white blood cells (WBCs). The tonsils trap and destroy infectious agents as they enter the body through the mouth. The lymphatic vessels circulate the lymph, and the lymph carries toxins and cellular waste products from the cell to the heart for filtration.

There is rapid growth of the thymus gland from birth to ten years. The action of the entire system declines from adulthood to old age, which means that the elderly are less able to respond to infection.

Respiratory
The respiratory system consists of the airway, lungs, and respiratory muscles. The airway is composed of the pharynx, larynx, trachea, bronchi, and bronchioles. The lungs contain air-filled sacs called alveoli, and they are covered by a visceral layer of double-layered pleural membrane. The intercostal muscles are located between the ribs, and the diaphragm—the largest muscle of the body—separates the thoracic cavity from the abdominal cavity.

On inspiration, the airway transports the outside air to the lungs, while the expired air carries the carbon dioxide that is removed by the lungs. The alveoli are the site of the exchange of carbon dioxide from the systemic circulation with the oxygen contained in the inspired air. The muscles help the thoracic cavity to expand and contract to allow for air exchange.

The respiratory rate in the infant gradually decreases from a normal of thirty to forty breaths per minute, until adolescence when it equals the normal adult rate of twelve to twenty breaths per minute. Pulmonary function declines after the age of sixty because the alveoli become larger and less efficient, and the respiratory muscles weaken.

Digestive
The digestive system includes the mouth, pharynx, esophagus, stomach, small intestine, large intestine, and sigmoid colon. The entire system forms a twenty-four-foot tube through which ingested food passes. Digestion begins in the mouth, where digestive enzymes are secreted in response to food intake. Food then passes through the esophagus to the stomach, which is a pouch-shaped organ that collects and holds food for a period of time. The small intestine begins at the distal end of the stomach. The lining of the small intestine contains many villi, which are small, hair-like projections that increase the absorption of nutrients from the ingested food. The large intestine originates at the distal end of the small intestine and terminates in the rectum. The large intestine is four feet long and has three segments, including the ascending colon along the right side, the transverse colon from right to left across the body, and the descending colon down the left side of the body, where the sigmoid colon begins.

The enzymes of the mouth, stomach, and the proximal end of the small intestine break down the ingested food into nutrients that can be absorbed and used by the body. The nutrients are absorbed by the small intestine. The large intestine removes the water from the waste products, which forms the stool. The muscle layer of the large intestine is responsible for peristalsis, which is the force that moves the waste products through the intestine.

The function of the digestive system declines more slowly than other body systems, and the changes that most often occur are the result of lifestyle issues or medication use.

Urinary
The urinary system includes the kidneys, ureters, bladder, and urethra. The kidneys are a pair of bean-shaped organs that lie just below and posterior to the liver in the peritoneal cavity. The nephron is the functional unit of the kidney, and there are about 1 million nephrons in each of the two kidneys. The ureters are hollow tubes that allow the urine formed in the kidneys to pass into the bladder. The urinary bladder is a hollow mucous lined pouch with the ureters entering the upper portion, and the urethra exiting from the bottom portion. The urethra is a tubular structure lined with mucous membrane that connects the bladder with the outside of the body.

In addition to the formation and excretion of the waste product urine, the nephron of the kidney also regulates fluid and electrolyte balance and contributes to the control of blood pressure. The ureters allow the urine to pass from the kidneys to the bladder. The bladder stores the urine and regulates the process of urination. The urethra delivers the urine from the bladder to the outside of the body.

The lifespan changes in the urinary system are more often the result of the effects of chronic disease on the system, rather than normal decline.

Reproductive
The major organs of the female reproductive organs include the uterus, cervix, vagina, ovaries, and fallopian tubes.

The uterus is a hollow, pear-shaped organ with a muscular layer that is positioned between the bladder and the rectum. The uterus terminates at the cervix, which opens into the vagina, which is open to the outside of the body. The ovaries, supported by several ligaments, are oval organs 1- to 2-inches long that are positioned on either side of the uterus in the pelvic cavity. The fallopian tubes, which are 4 inches long and .5 inches in diameter, connect the uterus with the ovaries.

The male reproductive organs include the penis, scrotum, testicles, vas deferens, seminal vesicles, and the prostate gland. In addition to the urethra, the penis contains three sections of erectile tissue. The scrotum is a fibromuscular pouch that contains the testes, the spermatic cord, and the epididymis. The pair of testes is suspended in the scrotum and each one is approximately 2 inches by 1 inch long. The vas deferens is a tubular pathway between the testes and the penis, and the seminal vesicles are small organs located between the bladder and the bowel. The prostate gland surrounds the proximal end of the urethra within the pelvic cavity.

The main function of the male reproductive system is the production of sperm. Unlike the female, beginning at puberty, several million immature sperm are produced every day in the testes. The sperm are transported through the vas deferens to the penis, and the prostate gland and seminal vesicles contribute fluids that support the activity of the sperm after ejaculation.

At puberty, egg maturation, menses, and sperm production begin, and the secondary sex characteristics appear. Female fertility declines at thirty years of age, and the maturation of eggs in the ovaries ceases at menopause, which occurs at fifty years of age. Sperm production continues from puberty until death; however, after sixty years of age the ability of the sperm to travel to the fallopian tube to fertilize an egg is decreased.

Endocrine
The glands of the endocrine system include the pituitary, thyroid, parathyroid, adrenal, and reproductive glands, as well as the hypothalamus, the pancreas, and the pineal body. The function of the system is to synthesize and secrete hormones that control body growth, sexual function, and

metabolism, which is the production and use of energy by the body. The thyroid gland, located on either side of the trachea, regulates energy production, or the rate at which the body uses ingested food to support body functions. The parathyroid, located on the upper margin of the thyroid gland, regulates calcium levels by the activation of Vitamin D, which increases intestinal absorption of calcium, and by regulating the amount of calcium that is stored in the bones or excreted by the kidneys. The adrenal glands, located on the upper margin of the kidneys, consist of the adrenal cortex and the adrenal medulla. The hormones secreted by the adrenal cortex are necessary for life and include: cortisol, or hydrocortisone, which regulates the breakdown of proteins, carbohydrates, and fats for energy production and the body's response to stress; corticosterone, which works with cortisol to regulate the immune system; and aldosterone, which contributes to blood-pressure control. The adrenal medulla secretions, including adrenaline, regulate the body's reaction to stress known as the fight-or-flight response. The ovaries secrete estrogen and the testes secrete testosterone, which regulate sexual maturation and function. The pancreas, located in the right upper quadrant of the abdomen, secretes the insulin that regulates blood sugar, in addition to other hormones that regulate water absorption and secretion in the intestines. The pineal gland, located in the center of the brain, secretes melatonin, which regulates the circadian rhythm or sleep cycle.

The nervous system connects each of these glands to the hypothalamus and the pituitary gland. The hypothalamus senses alterations in hormone secretions in all of these organs and conveys those messages to the pituitary gland, which then stimulates each specific organ to either increase or decrease secretion of the relevant hormone. This feedback system is necessary for homeostasis.

Sensory

The sensory organs include the eyes, ears, nose, tongue, and skin, and they contain special receptor cells that transmit information to the nervous system. The eyes receive and process light energy. The ears process sound waves and also contribute to the maintenance of equilibrium. The nose senses odors and the tongue senses taste. The skin responds to tactile stimulation, including pain, hot, cold, and touch. Internal organs also sense pain and pressure. The brain is responsible for processing all of these sensations.

The senses of touch and smell are active in the fetus and continue to mature after birth. Touch is especially important for infants. The elderly experience a decline in the acuity of all of the senses; however, eyesight and hearing are most commonly affected due to the effects of chronic diseases such as hypertension and diabetes.

Pathophysiology and Diseases of Body Systems

Integumentary

The function of the integumentary system may be affected by:

- Allergic responses, including eczema
- Infections resulting from bacteria, fungi, and viruses (herpes virus)
- Vasculature alterations, including venous stasis ulcers
- Genetic defects, including psoriasis
- Autoimmune disorders, including scleroderma
- Cancers, including basal cell, squamous cell, and melanoma

Musculoskeletal

The function of the musculoskeletal system may be affected by:

- Alterations in bine integrity, resulting in osteoporosis
- Fractures that result from injury or disease

Nervous

The function of the nervous system may be affected by:

- Acute injury, resulting in concussion and other catastrophic injuries
- Alterations in cognition, evidenced by Alzheimer's disease
- Alterations in movement, evidenced by Parkinson's disease
- Alterations in circulation, resulting in stroke
- Genetic defects, including Huntington's chorea
- Cancer, evidenced by brain tumors

Cardiovascular, hematopoietic, and lymphatic

The function of the cardiovascular system may be affected by:

- Decreased oxygen supply, resulting in myocardial infarction and angina
- Alterations in the blood vessels, resulting in hypertension

The function of the hematopoietic system may be affected by:

- Cancer, resulting in leukemia
- Alterations in red-blood-cell production, resulting in anemia

The function of the lymphatic system may be affected by:

- Cancer, resulting in lymphoma and Hodgkin's disease
- Infection

Respiratory

The function of the respiratory system may be affected by:

- Airway obstruction, resulting in chronic obstructive pulmonary disease (COPD) and emphysema
- Infections, resulting in pneumonia
- Allergic responses, resulting in asthma

Digestive

The function of the digestive system may be affected by:

- Inflammation, resulting in Crohn's disease and ulcerative colitis
- Autoimmune disease, evidenced by lupus erythematosus
- Cancer, resulting in colorectal tumor

<u>Urinary</u>
The function of the urinary system may be affected by:

- Infection, resulting in bladder infection and kidney infection
- Alterations in blood vessels, resulting in kidney failure
- Cancer

<u>Reproductive</u>
The function of the reproductive system may be affected by:

- Infection, resulting in vaginitis and prostatitis
- Genetic alterations, evidenced by sterility and endometriosis
- Cancer

<u>Endocrine</u>
The function of the endocrine system may be affected by:

- Alterations in metabolism, resulting in diabetes
- Alterations in fluid volume regulation, resulting in hypertension and Cushing's syndrome
- Cancer

<u>Sensory</u>
The function of the sensory system may be affected by:

- Alterations in perception, evidenced by deafness, blindness, and pain perception

Infection Control

Infectious Agents

Infectious agents can alter the function of any body system, and they stimulate the immune system.

- Bacteria are unicellular organisms that are either essential to normal body function or harmful to the body, and therefore capable of triggering an immune response.

- Viruses contain only a core of DNA or RNA and a protein coat. Common viruses include the flu viruses, acquired immune deficiency syndrome (AIDS), and chicken pox, which can lead to shingles.

- Fungi, which include yeasts and molds, are multicellular organisms that can cause local infections such as athlete's foot.

- Protozoa are single-celled parasites that can affect the lungs, skin, and gastrointestinal system. Manifestations and treatment are specific to the individual organisms.

- A parasite is any agent that lives in or on a host and causes harm to the host.

Modes of Transmission

- Direct contact requires skin-to-skin contact between an infected person and a host who is susceptible to the infectious agent.

- Indirect contact occurs when the susceptible host contacts an object that has been previously handled by the infected person.

- Airborne infections are spread through the movement of dust or from ventilation systems.

- Droplet infections occur from coughing and sneezing.

- The susceptible host may inhale infectious agents that are in the environment.

Infection Cycle/Chain of Infection

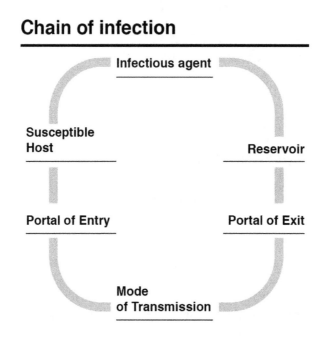

Chain of infection

Infectious agent

Susceptible Host

Reservoir

Portal of Entry

Portal of Exit

Mode of Transmission

In order to promote patient safety, the provider must be aware of the elements of the process or chain of infection, and employ all means necessary to prevent the transmission of the infectious agent. An infectious agent is any pathogen that is capable of transmitting an infection to a susceptible host. Once infected, the susceptible host becomes a reservoir for the infectious agent, where the agent is able to survive, grow, and multiply. The portal of exit is the route used by the infectious agent to move from a reservoir to another susceptible host. This route is often predicted by the body system that is affected by the pathogen; for example, the respiratory tract is often the portal of exit for influenza viruses. The mode of transmission identifies the manner by which the infectious agent makes contact with the host, and the provider must recognize that food, water, and insects are all possible modes of transmission, in addition to direct and indirect contact. The portal of entry is the host body system that serves as the initial point of contact with the infectious agent. The susceptible host is the individual who is infected by the pathogen, and the susceptibility to a given infectious agent will be influenced by genetics, immune function, and the individual's general health status at the point of contact.

Body's Natural Barriers

Along with the immune system, the skin, mucous membranes, tears, and stomach acids all act as natural barriers to inhibit the transmission of infectious agents.

Medical Asepsis

Medical asepsis is considered a "clean" technique that is aimed at reducing the number of infectious agents in a patient's environment.

Hand Hygiene

Hand hygiene is essential to maintaining medical asepsis. There are two acceptable methods: handwashing and the use of alcohol-based hand rubs.

All providers must wash their hands before and after patient contact, when handling any of the objects that enter the patient's environment, and when leaving the patient-care area.

Alcohol-based hand rubs are able to kill germs more effectively than soap and water and according to some authorities may be less irritating to the skin; however, soap and water are still the most effective when it comes to removing germs from the skin, though not necessarily killing them.

Sanitization

Sanitization is the process of cleaning utensils and the environment with soap and water to attain general cleanliness.

Disinfection

Disinfection refers to the use of more-potent cleaning agents to destroy infectious organisms, which exist on inanimate objects that exist in the patient-care environment.

Surgical Asepsis

Surgical asepsis is a process that eliminates any viable infectious agents from the immediate environment.

Surgical Scrub

Providers in the surgical suite will perform a surgical scrub, which is a handwashing technique aimed at reducing infectious agents to a minimum from the fingernails, hands, and forearms. The process involves a timed, five-minute systematic scrub with antimicrobial soap that begins with the hand and then progresses to the forearm. Once the scrub is complete, the hands are kept above the elbows to prevent contamination from areas of the body not included in the scrub. The provider then dries the skin thoroughly with a sterile towel.

Sterilization Techniques/Autoclave

Sterilization eliminates all transmissible organisms from inanimate objects. The autoclave is an efficient, cost-effective method of sterilization that utilizes moist heat to destroy organisms; however, it is not appropriate for heat-sensitive materials.

Before autoclaving, the provider will thoroughly clean all of the items to be processed and verify that all instruments are in the open position to ensure that all surfaces are exposed to the heat. The provider must be aware that different types of metals cannot be processed together, and carbon steel instruments must be wrapped in special towels to avoid the oxidation that can occur if the instruments come in contact with the stainless-steel trays of the autoclave.

To ensure sterility, the provider will include a sterilization indicator with each instrument or package.

Standard Precautions/Blood Borne Pathogen Standards

Standard precautions are standardized protocols that identify safe practices aimed at the prevention of infection by pathogens that exist in the blood and body fluids. These guidelines apply to all patients.

Body Fluids
With the exception of sweat, all body fluids are capable of transmitting an infectious agent from one source to another. The provider will observe all standard precautions for body fluids, including handwashing and the use of personal protective equipment consistent with the extent of estimated exposure to the body fluids. At a minimum, the provider will use gloves to handle contaminated articles, and to thoroughly clean or discard the items as appropriate.

Secretions
The provider will observe standard precautions for secretions and use a face shield or mask and eye shield to protect against the possibility of a droplet infection, as needed.

Excretions
As noted with secretions, the provider must treat all excretions as possible sources of infections, and comply with the mandatory handwashing and the use of gloves as the minimum protection.

Blood
Standard precautions for exposure to blood include special precautions for contamination by needle-stick injuries and contact with blood from other sources. In addition to handwashing, gloves, and eye protection, the provider will use venipuncture and injection systems that are equipped with safety features to protect against exposure to the blood.

Human Immunodeficiency Virus (HIV)-Human Papilloma Virus (HBV)-Hepatitis C (HCV)
Additional precautions are implemented for known transmissible infections such as HIV, HBV, and HCV. Transmission-based precautions include three   levels of protection, including contact, airborne, and droplet precautions. Patients must be in a protective environment that includes a private room with the appropriate air filtration system and dedicated patient-care items such as stethoscopes. Health care workers must use appropriate protective equipment and dispose of all contaminated care articles according to institutional policy.

Mucous Membranes
Appropriate precautions include the use of handwashing and gloves in addition to proper disposal of items that have been in contact with the mucous membranes.

Personal Protective Equipment
The purpose of personal protection equipment is to decrease the incidence of infection in health care workers. The equipment should be appropriate to the situation and degree of contamination. In addition, the equipment should be used consistently and correctly.

Gowns cover the entire body and have long sleeves that fit snugly around the wrists. Clean gowns may be used for patients in isolation, while sterile gowns are required for all invasive procedures. If contamination with fluids is anticipated, a fluid-repellent material should be chosen.

Gloves protect the hands and should be changed between individual tasks or if damaged to prevent cross contamination from one area to another area. Handwashing is also necessary after gloves are removed. Once gloves have been contaminated, they must be removed and discarded.

Masks must fit firmly over the bridge of the nose and the mouth. If contamination of other areas of the face is possible, as when irrigating wounds, a face shield that covers the entire face to the forehead is indicated. Specialized particulate masks must be used for airborne organisms such as tuberculosis.

Caps should fit snugly, covering the hair in order to protect the health care worker from contamination and to protect the patient during invasive procedures.

Eye protection from droplet infection and splashing of secretions cannot depend on personal eyeglasses or contact lenses. Depending on the anticipated contamination, a full shield may be chosen in the place of standard safety glasses and a mask.

Post-Exposure Plan
The post-exposure plan is a set of written guidelines that must be followed when a health care worker is exposed to an infectious pathogen as the result of a sharps injury, patient behavior, or failure of the personal protective equipment. The exact steps of the plan will be appropriate to the specific infectious agent. All exposures will be followed by a medical examination and serial laboratory tests to monitor for the presence of infection. Vaccinations aimed at limiting the incidence of disease may be appropriate in some circumstances. Individual institutions are responsible for educating all employees about the post-exposure plan, as well as monitoring the implementation of the plan following any incident that involves exposure of an employee to an infectious agent.

Biohazard Disposal/Regulated Waste

Biohazard waste is identified as any material that has been contaminated by body fluids or blood, which can potentially harm individuals or the environment. Disposal methods include the use of the incinerator, autoclave, or microwave in addition to chemical disinfection or irradiation. The disposal of biohazard waste is generally regulated by the Department of Health in the individual states, which means that health care workers must be aware of applicable state laws.

Sharps
Sharps include hypodermic needles, surgical scalpels, lancets, and all other devices that can puncture the intact skin. These devices may be destroyed by heat, oxidation of the stainless steel needles, or by passing an electrical current through the needles.

Blood and Body Fluids
Blood and body fluids are designated as biohazardous or medically regulated waste. At the bedside, these wastes are placed in the appropriate collection bags, which are identified as hazardous waste and subsequently destroyed by incineration.

Safety Data Sheets (SDS)
Safety data sheets contain detailed information for all substances that are designated as biohazardous, including the appropriate use of personal protective equipment, first aid protocols, and disposal requirements. Institutions are required to publish an SDS for any substance that is corrosive or may cause cancer, damage to an unborn fetus, or damage to the ovaries and testes.

Spill Kit
A spill kit contains all of the equipment and information that is necessary to safely clean an area after an accidental spill or leakage of a biohazardous material.

Patient Intake and Documentation of Care

Medical Record Documentation

Subjective Data
Subjective data is supplied by the patient.

- The *chief complaint* is the reason for the medical visit or hospital admission.

- The *present illness* is a detailed description of the symptoms related to the chief complaint.

- The *past medical history* identifies all of the patient's previous conditions and illnesses.

- The *family history* includes all diseases that have affected the patient's family. Genetically linked illnesses may be identified.

- The *social and occupational history* identifies lifestyle and work activities that may influence the patient's health, such as occupational exposure to biohazardous agents.

- The *review of systems* is a series of questions that are related to individual body organs or systems and identify the patient's specific concerns.

Objective Data
Objective data is observed by the provider. The data may be obtained through observation, physical assessment, or diagnostic testing.

Making Corrections
The process of making corrections in health care documentation must comply with agency policies. In general, the original text must remain visible with the erroneous information indicated with a single line through the text. The entry containing the revised information must be initialed and dated, and the use of "whiteout" and erasers is prohibited.

Treatment/Compliance
All treatments and the patient's compliance with those plans will be documented in the health history. This information is necessary for the evaluation of the effectiveness of the treatment plan.

Patient Preparation and Assisting the Provider

Vital Signs/Anthropometrics

<u>Blood Pressure</u>
Technique
To obtain an accurate measurement, the provider will:

- Assist the patient to a seated position.

- Expose the upper arm at the level of the heart.

- Apply the appropriately sized cuff.

- Palpate the antecubital space to identify the strongest pulsation point.

- Position the head of the stethoscope over the pulsation pulse.

- Slowly inflate the cuff to between 30 and 40 mm Hg above the patient's recorded blood pressure (BP). If this information is unavailable, the cuff may be inflated to between 160 and 180 mm Hg.

- Note the point at which the pulse is initially audible, which represents the systolic BP.

- Slowly deflate the cuff and record the point at which the pulse is initially audible as the systolic BP.

- Record the point at which the sounds are no longer audible as the diastolic BP.

Equipment
The *stethoscope* is a Y-shaped, hollow tube with earpieces and a diaphragm that transmits the sound to the earpieces when the provider places the diaphragm against the patient's body.

The *sphygmomanometer* includes the cuff, the mercury-filled gauge, or manometer that records the patient's pressure, and the release valve that regulates the air pressure in the cuff.

<u>Pulse</u>
Technique
To assess the pulse the provider will:

- Expose the intended pulse point.
- Palpate the area for the strongest pulsation.
- Position the middle three fingers of the hand on the point.
- Count the pulse for one full minute.

The provider will identify the pulse points that include the radial artery in the wrist, the brachial artery in the elbow, the carotid artery in the neck, the femoral artery in the groin, the popliteal artery behind the knee, and the dorsalis pedis and the posterior tibialis arteries in the foot.

The provider will assess the pulse rate by counting the number of pulsations per sixty minutes. In addition to the pulse rate, the provider will document the regularity or irregularity and strength of the pulsations.

Height/Weight/BMI
Technique
To record an accurate height, the provider must instruct the patient to:

- Remove all footwear.
- Stand straight with the back against the wall.
- Remain still until the height is recorded.

To record an accurate weight, the provider must first zero the scale and then instruct the patient to:

- Remove all heavy objects from the pockets.
- Stand on the scale facing forward.
- Remain still until the weight is recorded.

The BMI (body mass index) is equal to:

- Imperial English BMI Formula: $weight\ (lbs) \times 703 \div height\ (in^2)$
- Metric BMI Formula: $weight\ (kg) \div height(m^2)$

For example:

The BMI of a patient who weighs 150 pounds and is 5'6" is equal to:

$$\frac{150 \times 703}{66 \times 66} = \frac{105,450}{4,356} = 24.2 \text{ or } 24.0$$

Equipment
Body scales may be mechanical or digital. Some digital scales also provide detailed metabolic information including the BMI in addition to the weight. Other scales can accommodate patients who are confined to bed.

Body Temperature
There are five possible assessment sites for body temperature, including oral, axillary, rectal, tympanic, and temporal. The route will depend on the patient's age and the agency policies. Assessment of oral temperatures requires the provider to verify that the patient has had nothing to eat or drink for five minutes before testing in order to avoid inaccurate readings.

Thermometers may be digital with disposal covers for the probe, wand-like structures that use infrared technology and are moved across the forehead to the temporal area, or handles with disposable cones that measure the tympanic temperature.

Oxygen Saturation/Pulse Oximetry
When every hemoglobin molecule in the circulating blood volume is carrying the maximum number of four oxygen molecules, the oxygen saturation rate is 100 percent. The normal oxygen saturation level is 95 percent to 100 percent, and levels below 90 percent must be treated.

The provider measures oxygen saturation noninvasively by the application of a pulse oximetry device, which the provider will attach to the patient's finger. The device may be used for continuous or intermittent monitoring of the saturation rate.

The pulse oximeter is a foam-lined clip that attaches to the patient's finger and uses infrared technology to assess the oxygen saturation level, which is expressed as a percentage.

Respiration Rate
The respiratory rate is counted, and the breathing pattern is assessed. The provider should ensure that the patient is unaware that the breathing rate is being counted by leaving the fingers resting on the radial pulse site while the respiratory rate is assessed.

Recognize and Report Age-Specific Normal and Abnormal Vital Signs

Age	Temperature Degrees Fahrenheit	Pulse Range	Respiratory Rate Range	Blood Pressure mmHg
Newborns	98.2 axillary	100-160	30-50	75-100/50-70
0 - 5 years	99.9 rectal	80-120	20-30	80-110/50-80
6 - 10 years	98.6 oral	70-100	15-30	85-120/55-80
11 - 14 years	98.6 oral	60-105	12-20	95-140/60-90
15 - 20 years	98.6 oral	60-100	12-30	95-140/60-90
Adults	98.6 oral	50-80	16-20	120/80

Examinations

Methods
- *Auscultation* refers to listening to the sounds of body organs or processes, such as blood pressure, using a stethoscope.

- *Palpation* refers to using the hand or fingers to apply pressure to a body site to assess an organ for pain or consistency.

- *Percussion* refers to tapping on a body part to assess for rebound sounds. It may be used to assess the abdomen or the lungs.

- *Mensuration* refers to the measurement of body structures, such as measuring the circumference of the newborn's head.

- *Manipulation* refers to using the hands to correct a defect such as realigning the bones after a fracture.

- *Inspection* refers to the simple observation of the color, contour, or size of a body structure.

<u>Body Positions/Draping</u>
The provider will use proper draping to maximize the patient's privacy and to facilitate the planned procedures.

Draping Body Position

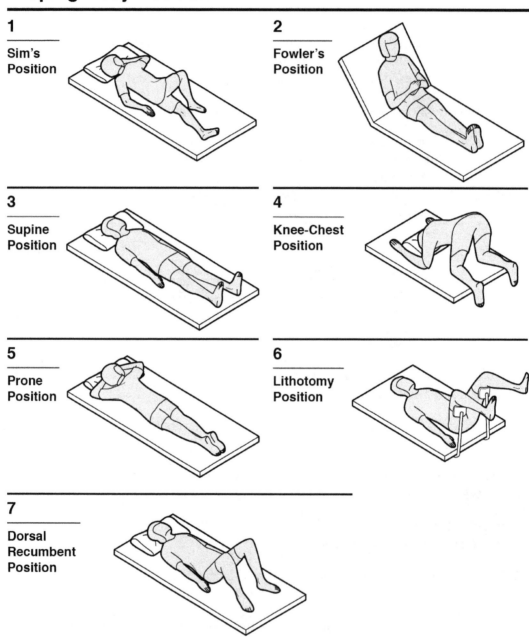

1
Sim's Position

2
Fowler's Position

3
Supine Position

4
Knee-Chest Position

5
Prone Position

6
Lithotomy Position

7
Dorsal Recumbent Position

<u>Pediatric Exam</u>
The purpose of the pediatric exam is to assess the child's growth and development and to provide family counseling regarding behavioral issues, nutrition, and injury protection. In addition, providers screen children for specific conditions at various ages to ensure that appropriate treatment is not delayed. For

instance, newborns are tested for phenylketonuria and hearing loss. Children between three and five years old are tested for alterations in vision, and school-aged children are screened for obesity.

Growth Chart
The growth chart is a systematic assessment of a child's growth pattern that can be compared to gender-specific norms.

Measurements
The head circumference, height, and body weight are measured in children from birth to three years of age. In children older than three, the BMI is measured in addition to height and weight.

The head circumference is measured from birth to three years of age. The provider will measure the head circumference by placing a flexible measuring tape around the widest circumference of the child's head, which most commonly is above the eyebrows and the top of the ears. The provider will weigh infants lying down without clothes or diapers, and older children on mechanical or digital scales. To assess an infant's height, the provider will lay the child on a flat surface with the knee straightened and extend the flexible tape from the top of the infant's head to the bottom of the foot. The provider will position older children with their backs to a wall for an accurate measurement of their height.

OB-GYN Exam
Pelvic Exam/ Papanicolaou (PAP) Smear

The pelvic exam is done to assess the organs of the female reproductive system. The ovaries and the uterus are assessed by palpation, and the cervix is assessed by inspection. The PAP smear sample is a screening test for cervical cancer. The sample, obtained from the opening of the cervix, is transferred to glass slides for processing.

Prenatal/Postpartum Exams
The provider performs the prenatal pelvic exam to assess the development of the fetus and the status of the maternal reproductive system. The pelvic exam is done at the first visit, but is not repeated with every visit. In a normal pregnancy, it may not be repeated until the third trimester. The provider performs the postpartum exam to assess the return of the maternal reproductive organs to the nonpregnant state.

Procedures

The provider will verify the order, identify the patient, and use proper handwashing technique and appropriate personal protective equipment for each of the following procedures.

Eye Irrigation
The purpose of the eye irrigation is to remove drainage or foreign bodies from the eye. The provider must be aware that alternative protocols are necessary for major trauma or exposure to toxic materials. The provider will instruct the   patient to perform frequent handwashing, refrain from touching the eye, report eye drainage/pain/alterations in vision, and avoid airborne contaminants.

The provider will assemble the necessary equipment, which includes the irrigating solution and syringe, sterile normal saline, appropriate personal protective equipment (PPE), a curved basin, and a waterproof towel.

The provider will assist the patient to a seated or supine position with the head turned to the affected side, and then position a waterproof towel under the patient's head. After removing any secretions from the eyelid and eyelashes with normal saline and gauze, the provider will use the nondominant hand to hold the eye open to expose the conjunctiva. The provider will position the curved basin against the patient's cheek and, holding the syringe tip at least 1 inch from the eye, irrigate the eye from the inner to the outer canthus. Once the eye is free of all drainage, the provider will dry the area with sterile gauze and adhere a protective covering, if ordered. The provider will assist the patient to a position of comfort and document the procedure.

Ear Irrigation

The purpose of the ear irrigation is to remove impacted cerumen or small foreign bodies from the ear.

The provider will instruct the patient to refrain from inserting anything into the ear, to report drainage/pain/alterations in hearing, and to use a washcloth to clean the outer ear.

The provider will assemble the necessary equipment, which includes the irrigating syringe, sterile normal saline warmed to body temperature, appropriate PPE, a curved basin, cotton balls, and a waterproof towel.

The provider will assist the patient to a seated or supine position with the head turned to the affected side, and then position a waterproof towel under the patient's head. After positioning the curved basin against the side of the head, the provider will remove secretions from the outer ear and pinna with normal saline and gauze. To expose the auditory canal in infants, the provider will pull the pinna down and to the rear of the head, and in older children and adults the provider will pull the pinna up and to the rear of the head. After verifying that the canal is not occluded by the syringe tip, the provider will direct the flow of the solution to the top of the canal and allow the irrigating fluid to flow back into the basin. Once all secretions have been removed, the provider will dry the area with gauze and loosely insert a cotton ball to absorb any additional drainage. The provider will then assist the patient to lie on the affected side to promote drainage and document the procedure.

Dressing Change

The purpose of the dressing change is to assess the wound, remove drainage, and promote healing. The provider will instruct the patient to report increased pain, drainage, or odor.

The provider will assemble the necessary equipment, which includes sterile normal saline, sterile dressing supplies, waterproof pads, and the appropriate PPE.

The provider will provide pain medication for the patient thirty minutes before the procedure as appropriate. The provider will place a waterproof pad under the patient, expose the wound, and remove the existing dressing. The provider will then clean the wound with sterile gauze and NS by wiping from the center of the wound to the outer edge, gently dry the clean wound with sterile gauze, and apply the new dressing. After the dressing is secured, the provider will record the condition of the wound, the amount and character of the drainage, and the patient's response to the procedure.

Suture/Staple Removal

The purpose of the procedure is to remove the suture materials from a healing wound.

The provider will instruct the patient to report any drainage, increased pain, or fever, and to keep the wound clean. If steri-strips are ordered to secure the wound after the removal of the staples/sutures, the provider will instruct the patient to leave them in place because they will gradually separate from the skin seven to ten days after application.

The provider will gather the necessary equipment that includes sterile normal saline, sterile gauze, staple/suture removal kit, sterile gloves, appropriate PPE, and waterproof pads.

The provider will expose the wound, remove the existing dressing, clean the wound as ordered, and assess the integrity of the incision. The provider will begin at one end of the incision, removing only every other staple/suture initially, by inserting the tip of the removal instrument between the skin and the staple, and gently closing the instrument, which will force the edges of the staple up and out of the wound (see image below). To remove the sutures, the provider will use forceps to pick up the free thread of the suture to raise the suture material above the surface of the skin, and then insert the blade of the scissors (the blade with the circular depression) under the suture material to cut the suture (see image below). Once the integrity of the wound is verified, the provider will remove the remaining staples/sutures, apply steri-strips as ordered, and document the procedure and the condition of the wound.

Staple in Place

Removed Staple

Forceps

99

Sterile Procedures

Surgical Assisting

Surgical assisting refers to the procedures in the surgical suite that may be assigned to certified assistants. Some of these activities include suturing, suctioning, clearing the operative field of blood, and maintaining traction on retractors.

Surgical Tray Prep

Surgical tray prep is the collection and preparation of all of the surgical instruments and equipment necessary for a specific surgical procedure performed by a specific surgical team.

Antiseptic Skin Prep

The antiseptic skin prep is required to remove all possible organisms and debris from the surgical site and to prevent contamination of the wound or postoperative infection. The provider washes the skin with soap and water to remove any dirt and debris, and then applies bacteriocidal agents according to agency policy.

Sterile Field Boundaries

Sterile field boundaries relate to the operative field, the surgical staff, and the operative instruments. The boundaries of the operative field include the surgical site and the proximal areas of the sterile drapes. All members of the surgical team are dressed in sterile gowns, sterile gloves with appropriate masks, eye protection, and head coverings; however, once a member of the team approaches the operative site, only the front of the gown from the waist to the mid chest and the arms to the elbows is considered sterile. In addition, only the inside of the sterile packaging for instruments is considered sterile.

Surgical Instruments:

Classification	Instrument Use
Cutting/Grinding/Dissecting	Remove by cutting with scissors or a knife Smooth irregular surfaces in bone Remove tissue from the body
Clamping	Control blood loss Bypass blood flow from the surgical site
Grasping/Holding	Move structures to gain access to surgical site Stabilize structures for dissection
Probing	Assess distal anatomy
Dilating/Enlarging	Restore anatomical lumen Increase access to the operative site
Retracting	Increase visibility of the operative site by displacing adjacent organs
Suctioning	Maintain surgical site, free of excess fluid Remove surgical debris and irrigation fluid

Patient Education/Health Coach

Health Maintenance and Disease Prevention

Diabetic Teaching and Home Care

Diabetic teaching and home care: Prior to discharge, the patient will participate in a comprehensive program in order to learn about diabetes, self-care for diabetes, and the process of home monitoring.

Home blood sugar monitoring provides improved control of the patient's blood by more frequent assessment of the blood glucose level and more timely intervention of abnormal levels. The provider will assess the patient's ability to follow the treatment plan.

Patient Mobility Equipment and Assistive Devices
The provider must instruct the patient on the proper use of patient mobility equipment and assistive devices. Depending on the specific injury or condition, the patient may use assistive devices such as crutches, walkers, or canes to maintain mobility during the recovery period or for longer periods of time. Patients must receive appropriate safety instruction in the correct use of any device in order to maintain safety.

Pre-/Post-Op Care Instructions
Pre-/post-op care instructions are designed to minimize preoperative surgical delays and complications and to promote the patient's recovery following discharge. Providers, commonly advanced practice nurses, conduct preoperative assessments and educational sessions, while community-based nurses provide care once the patient is discharged.

Patient-Administered Medications
Patient-administered medications are those medications that are self-administered. The provider must assess the patient's ability to comprehend the details of the medication information and safe administration and provide resources to ensure the patient's ongoing safety.

Home Blood-Pressure Monitoring
The research relevant to the use of home blood-pressure monitoring systems indicates that patients who closely monitor their blood-pressure readings are better able to control the lifestyle factors associated with hypertension. Some of these lifestyle factors include dietary intake of salt, smoking behavior, and participation in aerobic exercise.

Home Anticoagulation Monitoring
Home anticoagulation testing is important to the consistent control of blood values. Recent advances even provide Bluetooth transmission of testing results directly to health care providers. This timely reporting also equates to better and safer control of the anticoagulant plan.

Home Cholesterol Monitoring
Home cholesterol monitoring is most effective in influencing lifestyle decisions related to diet, because the values do not change rapidly and, therefore, dosages are not frequently revised.

Alternative Medicine
Alternative medicine includes complementary treatments that may not be offered by health care providers, including massage, acupuncture, herbs, meditation, and homeopathy.

Wellness/Preventive Care

Cancer Screening
Cancer screening tests relevant to several organ systems have effectively decreased the incidence and mortality of cancer in those systems. Common screening tests include the PAP test for cervical cancer, colonoscopy for colon cancer, and mammography for breast cancer. Recently, screening for lung cancer with advanced computed tomography (CT) technology in patients with a history of smoking has been proposed, in an effort to identify lung cancers at an earlier stage that may be treated more successfully. Conversely, the research indicates that there is insufficient evidence to support any relationship

between decreased disease incidence and morbidity and the prostate-specific antigen test (PSA) measurements for prostate cancer, or the annual full-body skin assessments by a dermatologist. In addition, there are no screening tests available for ovarian cancer.

Sexually Transmitted Infections
Sexually transmitted diseases, including chancroid, chlamydia, genital herpes, gonorrhea, hepatitis C, HIV, and syphilis, are caused by intimate contact. The scope of treatment ranges from oral antibiotics for chlamydia to long-term antiviral treatment for HIV and hepatitis C infections. Complications are common when the initial infection is not treated.

Hygienic Practices
Hygienic practices can reduce the spread of an infectious agent from one source to another.

Hand Washing
Handwashing is effective in decreasing the transmission of infectious agents from one person to another person or object, as long as it is correctly and consistently performed.

Cough Etiquette
Cough etiquette requires that an individual cover the mouth and nose when coughing to prevent the spread of infection by droplet contact.

Smoking Risks and Cessation
Smoking by direct contact or through secondhand exposure can result in lung cancer and other obstructive lungs diseases such as COPD and emphysema. Smoking cessation programs are offered by many private and governmental agencies, and providers monitor the use of prescription medications that assist with cessation efforts.

Recognition of Substance Abuse
Abuse of recreational or prescription drugs may be evidenced by changes in behavior, appetite, and sleep patterns. Affected students may neglect course work and ignore family responsibilities. Providers work with parents and educators to identify at-risk individuals.

Osteoporosis Screening/Bone-Density Scan
Osteoporosis is the "thinning" of the bone, which most commonly affects postmenopausal women. The degree and progression of the changes associated with osteoporosis can be measured by the bone-density exam, which compares a patient's test results with the results of younger patients who are disease free.

Domestic Violence Screening and Detection
The efficiency of domestic violence screening and detection is often hampered by the reluctance of the abused individual to report the abuse. Institutions and insurance companies have included routine assessment questions related to a patient's perceptions of personal safety; however, the widespread acceptance and effectiveness of these measures are not known.

Nutrition

Basic Principles

<u>Food Nutrients</u>
Carbohydrates
Carbohydrates are organic (containing carbon) compounds that are converted into energy for the body. They may be simple, such as refined table sugar, or complex, such as pasta, rice, and fiber.

Fats
Fats are lipid-containing compounds that are necessary for cell wall integrity, energy storage, and protection of all body organs against injury. Cholesterol is a body fat that exists in two forms: low-density lipoprotein (LDL) and high-density lipoprotein (HDL). LDLs are associated with the formation and progression of atherosclerosis, which is a build-up of lipid cells in the vasculature that results in hypertension and cardiovascular disease. Fats are also classified by the configuration of the hydrogen bonds and are classified as saturated fats, which are solid at room temperature, or unsaturated fats, which are liquid at room temperature. Research indicates that replacing saturated fats with unsaturated fats in the diet facilitates the removal of excess cholesterol from the body. Fats are contained in dairy and animal products, nuts, and vegetable oils. Current recommendations include a consuming a balanced diet that provides unsaturated fats and limited animal fats.

Proteins
Proteins are also organic compounds that contain carbon, hydrogen, and oxygen and form amino acids, the building blocks of the protein molecule. There are nine essential amino acids that must be consumed because the body cannot synthesize them. A complete protein consists of all nine essential amino acids, while an incomplete protein is deficient in one or more of the essential amino acids. Proteins are essential for all intracellular processes and as enzymes that facilitate all chemical reactions in the body. Nutritional sources of protein include animal products, dairy products, beans, and tofu.

Minerals/Electrolytes
Mineral/electrolytes are metals and nonmetals, including sodium, potassium, chloride, phosphorous, magnesium, calcium, and sulfur. They are necessary for fluid balance, transmission of nervous impulses, bone maintenance, blood clotting, healthy teeth, and protein synthesis and cardiac-impulse conduction. Minerals and electrolytes are generally consumed in adequate amounts from a balanced diet.

Vitamins
Vitamins are organic compounds that are necessary for blood clotting, immune function, maintenance of teeth, and the action of enzymes. There are two classes of vitamins. Fat-soluble vitamins, including A, D, E, and K, can be stored in excess in the body in the event of excessive intake. Water-soluble vitamins, including B-complex and C, are not stored in the body and ingested amounts greater than body requirements will be excreted in the urine. Vitamins are present in fruits, vegetables, fish, organ meats, and dairy.

Fiber
Dietary fiber is composed of complex carbohydrates and other plant substances that are not broken down by the digestive enzymes. Fiber can be water soluble or insoluble, and both forms contribute to the normal function of the gastrointestinal system. Soluble fiber that is present in oatmeal, blueberries, nuts, and beans facilitates the excretion of cholesterol, controls abrupt increases in blood glucose levels, and contributes to normal bowel function. The insoluble fiber that is present in whole grains, the skin

and seeds of many fruits, and brown rice improves bowel function and also contributes to a feeling of fullness following food intake, which can lead to modest weight loss.

Water
Making up about 75 percent of the body, water is a vital necessity to human life. Water feeds cells and organs, creates a lubricant around the joints, and regulates body temperature. It is also important to digestion, as water moves food through the intestines.

Dietary Supplements
Dietary supplements contain various nutrients that are intended to compensate for inadequate dietary intake of those elements. These products should be used with care by anyone who also takes prescription medications because adverse interactions between the two are common.

Special Dietary Needs

Weight Control
Weight control requires a balanced diet that is calorie controlled and combined with adequate aerobic exercise. Current research indicates that the consumption of sugar and white flour, rather than dietary fats, is the greatest dietary threat to successful weight management.

Diabetes
Diabetes requires a balanced diet that is carbohydrate controlled. Diabetes may be due to a lack of insulin production by the pancreas or cellular insensitivity to the insulin that is present in the bloodstream. The controlled intake of carbohydrates limits the amount of insulin that is necessary to protect the body against the side effects of chronically elevated blood glucose levels.

Cardiovascular Disease
Cardiovascular disease most often is accompanied by excess fluid volume that is manifested by hypertension and edema. The condition requires a balanced diet that is sodium controlled, with adequate fluid intake.

Hypertension
Hypertension is associated with fluid volume excess, which means that excess dietary sodium and fluid should be avoided.

Cancer
Cancer may affect multiple body systems, which means that the diet should be balanced with additional calories to meet energy needs.

Lactose Sensitivity/Intolerance
Lactose sensitivity/intolerance results from the deficiency of the enzyme lactase, which is necessary for the breakdown or digestion of lactose, a sugar found in dairy products. This deficiency can result in stomach bloating, nausea, vomiting, and diarrhea following the ingestion of dairy products.

Gluten Free
Gluten-free diets must be free of wheat, barley, and rye in any form. This means that, in addition to bread, all processed foods must be avoided. Gluten intolerance may be a symptom of celiac disease, which affects the absorption of food in the small intestine, or an allergic response to wheat gluten; however, it is most commonly due to the lack of a necessary digestive enzyme. Possible manifestations include stomach bloating, diarrhea, fatigue, and weight loss.

Food Allergies

Food allergies can be related to one or several foods for a given patient. The allergic responses can range from mild to life threatening. The diet must be balanced and free of the allergens.

Eating Disorders

Eating disorders are psychologically induced alterations in nutrition. The most common disorders include anorexia nervosa, bulimia, and binge-eating disorder. Anorexia nervosa is seen most commonly in young women and is manifested by a fear of gaining weight and refusal to eat. The effects of this self-imposed starvation can vary from mild nutritional deficits to cardiac failure and death. Bulimia is also related to the fear of gaining weight and is manifested by the intake of large amounts of food followed by self-induced vomiting or purging, fasting, and depression. Bulimic patients can sustain significant damage to the mouth and teeth as a result of the effects of gastric acids associated with the vomiting. Binge eating occurs in men and women and is manifested by the regular episodes of the consumption of large amounts of food that are followed by feelings of depression. These individuals are often obese and relate these episodes to being out of control. In general, these diseases are difficult to resolve, and relapses are common.

Collecting and Processing Specimens

Methods of Collection

Blood
For a venipuncture process, the provider will:

- Identify the patient, review the order, and label the collection tubes.
- Assess the nondominant hand to identify a vein that is straight and palpable.
- Wash hands and apply PPE.
- Clean the selected site with an alcohol swab per agency policy.
- Inspect the test-specific vacuum tubes and needles to verify that:
    - The tube is securely sealed and vacuum has been maintained.
    - Appropriate additives such anticoagulants or other fixatives that may be required to maintain the sample are present in the tube.
    - The chosen needle size is appropriate to the selected vein.
- Complete the venipuncture per agency policy.
- Apply pressure and a sterile dressing to the venipuncture site.
- Submit the sample for processing per agency policy.

The provider will use a capillary/dermal puncture to obtain blood from small children or when only a small volume of blood is necessary as in finger-stick puncture for blood glucose analysis.

Urine
The provider can collect a random urinalysis any time the patient voids.

To obtain a midstream/clean catch urine sample, the provider will instruct the patient to first clean the urinary meatus with the appropriate antiseptic solution, void without collecting the initial volume, and then deposit the remaining output into the container.

Before beginning the collection of a timed twenty-four-hour collection, the provider must obtain a storage container containing any necessary preservative from the laboratory, and confirm the accommodations for refrigeration of the sample if required. The first time the patient voids, the provider will discard the specimen and record the time. All urine collected in the following twenty-four-hour period will be collected by the provider and stored in the prepared container at the prescribed temperature.

Catheterization may be used to obtain a sterile specimen. The provider will pass the sterile catheter into the bladder to drain the urine into a sterile container, which must then be labeled and transported to the lab according to agency policy.

The pediatric urine collector is a plastic pouch attached to a foam adhesive backed base. The provider will verify that the skin around the urinary meatus is clean, dry, and free of powder or lotions. The provider will adhere the adhesive section of the collection device over the urinary meatus and replace the patient's diaper.

Fecal Specimen
The provider will place the fecal specimen in a clean, leak-proof, properly labeled container, and promptly transport the sample to the laboratory for processing.

Sputum Specimen
The sputum specimen must contain sputum, not saliva, and it is best obtained early in the morning.

Swabs
The provider will verify the order, identify the patient, and use proper handwashing technique and appropriate personal protective equipment for each of the following procedures.

Throat Swab
After assisting the patient to a seated position in a chair or bed, the provider will use sterile swabs to remove the sample from the back of the throat while avoiding contact with the uvula and tongue. The provider will then break the tips of the swabs and secure them in the labeled collection sleeve, transport the sample to the lab according to agency policy, and document the sample collection time and site.

Genital
The provider will position the patient according to the site being sampled. The provider will use sterile swabs to sample the top of the vaginal vault for a vaginal swab, the center of the cervical os for a cervical swab, or the urinary meatus for a urethral swab. The provider will then break the tips of the swabs and secure them in the labeled collection sleeve, transport the sample to the lab according to agency policy, and document the sample collection time and site.

Wound
The provider will position the patient according to the site being sampled. The provider will remove and discard the existing dressing, use sterile swabs to obtain the sample from the center of the wound, then break the tips of the swabs and secure them in the labeled collection sleeve. Once the swabs are secured, the provider will dress the wound, ensure that the sample is delivered to the laboratory, and document the wound assessment and the sample collection time and site.

Nasopharyngeal
The provider will position the patient in a seated position with the head tilted back. After verifying the patency of the nares, the provider will insert the sterile swab 3 to 4 inches into the nasopharynx, rotate

the swaps to obtain the sample, remove the swabs, break the tips of the swabs to secure them in the labeled collection sleeve, transport the specimen to the laboratory, and document the collection site and time.

Prepare, Process, and Examine Specimens

Proper Labeling
Provider errors related to specimen collection are a threat to patient safety. Most recently, the use of two patient-specific identifiers has been mandated as the standard for all patient specimens. The provider must verify the patient's name and date of birth or other unique identifier per agency policy for all specimens that are submitted for processing.

Sources of Contamination
Collected samples may be contamination by extraneous body secretions and other environmental debris or infectious agents. Deviations in sterile technique are also a possible source of specimen contamination.

Specimen Preservation
The provider should be aware of all conditional requirements for the collection of a particular specimen.

Refrigeration
Samples collected over an extended period of time, such as twenty-four-hour urine collections or fecal samples may require a dedicated refrigeration source for the duration of the testing period. In general, most culture specimens must be refrigerated if there is an anticipated delay in processing; however, culture samples of cerebrospinal fluid and blood must be processed without delay, and should not be refrigerated.

Fixative
Fixatives are chemical substances that are added to preserve test specimens for processing. The solutions are specific to the type of testing, which means that histological testing of tissue biopsies may require different fixative solutions than chemistry testing of venous blood. The provider must be certain that all laboratory requirements are met for specimen collection and submission.

Recordkeeping
Laboratory personnel must verify that all data related to the ordering, collecting, and reporting of laboratory testing is appropriately documented in the electronic health record (EHR) and laboratory logbooks in accordance with agency policies.

Incubator
An incubator, a closed device that is atmospherically controlled with respect to a controlled environment, is essential for the growth and maintenance of cell cultures and microbial cultures.

Centrifuge
The centrifuge is a laboratory device that rapidly spins samples, which results in the separation of the less dense elements from the heavier elements according to the sedimentation principle. The process of differential centrifugation can separate cellular organelles from the individual cell, while isopycnic centrifugation can be used to isolate DNA strands. Sucrose gradient centrifugation can be used to refine viruses and other small cellular inclusions.

Microscope

A microscope is used to view substances, structures, or organisms that are not visible without magnification. The optical or light microscope, the first to be developed, uses light and a series of lenses to magnify an image up to four hundred times the actual size. The electron microscope aims a beam of high-speed electrons at a sample, which interacts with the sample to form an image. The scanning electron microscope interacts with the surface of the sample, while the transmission electron microscope interacts with the full thickness of the sample in order to produce an image. Electron microscopes can magnify a structure up to 10 million times the actual size.

Inoculating a Culture

Inoculating a culture is the process of transferring a specimen to a culture medium by using an inoculating loop, which the provider uses to disperse that sample in a streaking motion back and forth across the media plate. Alternatively, the provider can add the sample to test tubes that contain the media.

Microbiologic Slides

The microbiologic slides are pieces of glass that provide the base for microscopic samples. A dry mount refers to a sample placed on a slide with a cover slip. A wet mount slide contains a sample that is suspended in a small amount of liquid—such as water or glycerin—to increase the refraction of the light, and a cover slip.

Quality Control/Quality Assurance

Testing protocols are test-specific, standardized instructions for laboratory processes.

The provider will retain all testing records for completed laboratory analyses, which may be used to measure the degree of consistency with control values. Daily performance logs track the personnel completing the analyses and the test results on a daily basis.

All laboratory personnel are required to meet all manufacturer requirements for daily equipment maintenance protocols for laboratory instruments, in addition to documenting those activities in the maintenance log.

All laboratory personnel are responsible for conducting and documenting the calibration or verification of the quantitative measurement of all instruments.

Daily control testing refers to the daily process of comparing random testing results to a control.

All laboratory personnel must monitor temperature controls to prevent the destruction of collected specimens due to the effects of alterations in temperature on the specimen or lab chemicals.

Reagent storage refers to the maintenance of laboratory reagents within the proper temperature range. Reagents are most commonly maintained in cold storage or frozen.

Tests waved by the Clinical Laboratory Improvement Amendments (CLIA) as identified by the Food and Drug Administration (FDA) are a group of tests that are cleared for home use and in health care agencies that have a certificate of waiver and a documented quality assurance plan. Health care agencies that hold certificates of waiver for testing will be subject to periodic evaluations. In addition, nonclinical community agencies may apply for a certificate for waived rapid HIV testing or work with a clinical site that has a certificate of waiver for the test. The waived tests include only tests that are technically simple to perform and carry a low risk of harm to the patient even if they are performed incorrectly. Common waived-test categories identified in the list of more than 1,400 test systems include:

- Drug abuse screening.
- Ovulation calculation.
- Pregnancy.
- HIV.
- Electrolytes and liver function.
- Blood glucose.
- Fecal occult blood.
- Cholesterol and lipid profile.
- Lyme disease.
- Basic metabolic panel including calcium.

Laboratory Panels and Performing Selected Tests

Urinalysis
- Physical: The provider will perform a visual assessment of the color and turbidity of the urine sample.

- Chemical: The provider will use the reagent strip to assess the specific gravity, the pH, and the presence and quantity of protein, glucose, ketones hemoglobin and myoglobin, leukocyte esterase, bilirubin, and urobilirubin.

- Microscopic: The provider will separate the urine sediment from the fluid volume to microscopically identify the presence of RBCs, WBCs, epithelial cells, bacteria, yeasts, and parasites.

- Culture: The provider will assess the presence of infectious agents in the urine sample by inoculating the agar plates, incubating sample at body temperature, and observing, and documenting any growth at twenty-four and forty-eight hours after inoculation of the sample.

Hematology Panel
- Hematocrit (HCT): The provider will assess the RBC count as defined by the hematocrit by placing the anticoagulated blood sample into the microhematocrit centrifuge and documenting the results.

- Hemoglobin: The provider will assess the amount of the hemoglobin protein that is present in the red blood cells by placing the anticoagulated blood sample into the microhematocrit centrifuge and documenting the results.

- Erythrocyte Sedimentation Rate (ESR): The provider will assess the ESR, which is a nonspecific indicator of inflammation, by placing the anticoagulated sample in the Westergren tube and recording the height of the settled RBCs after one hour.

- Automated Cell Counts: The provider will use the automated device to assess RBC, WBC, and platelet counts by preparing the sample, obtaining, and documenting the results.

- Coagulation testing/international normalized ratio (INR): The provider will calculate the INR, which is used to assess blood-clotting levels in patients being treated with Warfarin, according to laboratory protocol after verifying that the sample was not drawn from a heparinized line.

<u>Chemistry/Metabolic Testing</u>
Glucose
The provider will identify the blood glucose sample, which measures the amount glucose in the circulating blood volume, as fasting or nonfasting before processing and documenting the results.

Kidney Function Tests
Kidney function is assessed by measuring the levels of metabolic waste products, including blood urea nitrogen (BUN) and creatinine, and by calculating the glomerular filtration rate (GFR), which corresponds with the clearance of waste products from the blood by the kidneys. The provider will process the sample to obtain the BUN and creatinine levels. The provider will then use the creatinine level and the patient's age, body size, and gender to calculate to the GFR according to the agency-approved equation for GFR. There are four equations that may be used to calculate the GFR in adults that include the Modification of Diet in Renal Disease (MDRD), the Study equation (IDMS-traceable version), and the Chronic Kidney Disease Epidemiology Collaboration (CKD-EPI) equation.

Liver Function Tests
Elevated levels of alanine transaminase (ALT) and aspartate aminotransferase (AST), two liver enzymes, indicate acute/chronic hepatitis, cirrhosis, or liver cancer. Decreased levels of these enzymes may be due to Vitamin B-12 deficiency. Albumin, a protein synthesized by the liver that is necessary for the maintenance of osmotic pressure in the vasculature, is decreased in liver failure due to cirrhosis or cancer. The liver processes bilirubin, a waste product resulting from the normal destruction of old red blood cells, for excretion by the gastrointestinal system; however, elevated levels may be due to liver failure or transfusion reactions. The provider will verify a ten-minute centrifuge time, process the sample, and document results.

Lipid Profile
Excess dietary intact of animal fats can result in elevated total cholesterol and low-density lipoprotein (LDL) or "bad cholesterol" levels, while elevated high-density lipoprotein (HDL) or "good cholesterol" levels are the result of appropriate nutrition or the effect of cholesterol-lowering medications. Elevated triglycerides levels may result from diabetes, obesity, liver failure, or kidney disease. The provider will verify that the fasting sample was obtained before the administration of N-Acetylcysteine (NAC) or Metamizole, if indicated. The provider will then process the sample per protocol within two hours of the venipuncture and document the results.

Hemoglobin A1c
Hemoglobin A1c measures the percentage of the hemoglobin molecules that are coated or glycated with glucose. The hemoglobin molecules are located in the red blood cell, which has a lifespan of 110 to 120 days; therefore, the hemoglobin A1c test measures the average blood sugar for a four-month period. The normal A1c level is less than 5.7 percent; levels between 5.7 percent and 6.4 percent indicate prediabetes and levels greater than 6.5 percent indicate diabetes. Elevated HGB A1c levels must be confirmed with additional testing before treatment is initiated. The provider will inform the patient that fasting is not required, process the sample, and document results.

Immunology

Mononucleosis Test

The immune system produces heterophile proteins in response to the presence of the Epstein-Barr virus (EBV), the causative agent of mononucleosis. Specific tests include the analysis of the viral capsid antigen (VCA), the early antigen (EA), or the EBV nuclear antigen (EBNA). The Monospot test detects antibodies that are not specific for mononucleosis, leading to false positive and false negative results. In addition, the Monospot test may be insensitive to the heterophile antibodies produced by children with mononucleosis. The provider will freeze the sample if processing is delayed beyond twenty-four hours after preparation.

Rapid Group A Streptococcus Test

Identification of the beta-hemolytic bacterium **Streptococcus pyogenes**, the most common cause of acute pharyngitis in adults and children, is obtained by using isothermal nucleic acid amplification technology. The provider will transfer the sample to the testing device adhering to proper wait-times, process the sample, and document the results.

C-Reactive Protein (CRP)

CRP is an indicator of inflammation that is released into the bloodstream in response to tissue injury or the onset of an infection. The provider will verify that all reagents and the serum sample are at room temperature, assess the processed sample for agglutination, and document the results.

HCG Pregnancy Test

Serum levels of human chorionic gonadotropin hormone detect the presence of a pregnancy. Elevated levels may indicate a normal pregnancy, either single or multiple, chorionic cancer, or hydatiform mole. The provider will centrifuge the clotted sample for ten minutes at room temperature, and document the results.

H. pylori

There are three testing methods for the *Helicobacter pylori* organism, including histological examination and culture of samples obtained by endoscopic biopsy, the urea breath test (UBT) that measures CO_2 levels on exhalation, and the fecal antigen test that identifies antibodies to the organism. The provider will verify that patient has avoided antibiotics and bismuth preparations for two weeks prior to the testing. The provider will process all samples according to the specific test requirements and document the results.

Influenza

Influenza testing methods include the Rapid Influenza Diagnostic Test (RIDT), and the Real Time Polymerase Chain Reaction, and the viral culture, which identify the genetic material of the virus in secretions obtained from a nasal or throat swab. The provider will process all samples according to the specific test requirements and document the results.

Fecal Occult Blood Testing

Occult bleeding is not visibly apparent, which means that detection methods rely on the chemical reaction between the blood and the testing reagents for identification of blood in a sample. For home sample collection with guaiac testing, the provider will instruct the patient to collect three samples on three different days to optimize results. The patient will secure the test card and submit it to the provider for testing. The provider will apply a guaiac solution to the sample to identify a bluish tinge in the test area, which is considered positive for the presence of occult blood.

Diagnostic Testing

Cardiovascular Tests

<u>Electrocardiography (EGG/ECG)</u>
To perform a standard 12-lead EGG/ECG, the provider will:
- Verify the order and obtain all equipment before approaching the patient.
- Explain the procedure to the patient and assist him/her to a supine position.
- Expose the limbs and the chest, maintaining appropriate draping to preserve patient's privacy.
- Clean the electrode sites with alcohol and remove excess body hair according to agency policy.
- Attach electrodes to appropriate anatomical positions.
- Attach machine cables to the electrodes.
- Enter the patient data and calibrate the machine as necessary.
- Request that the patient does not move or speak.
- Obtain an artifact-free tracing.
- Remove the electrodes and residual conductive gel.
- Return the patient to a position of comfort.
- Submit the tracing for interpretation.

Correct Placement of EKG Leads
The accuracy of the tracing is dependent on correct lead placement; therefore, the provider will position the chest leads as follows:

- V_1 - right sternal border at the level of the fourth intercostal space
- V_2 - left sternal border at the level of fourth intercostal space
- V_3 - centered between V_2 and V_4
- V_4 - the midclavicular line at the level of the fifth intercostal space
- V_5 - horizontal to V_4 at the anterior axillary line
- V_6 - horizontal to V_4 at the midaxillary line

The provider must attach the limb leads to the extremities, not the torso. In addition, the provider must avoid large muscle groups, areas of adipose tissue deposit, and bony prominences when placing the limb leads on the four extremities.

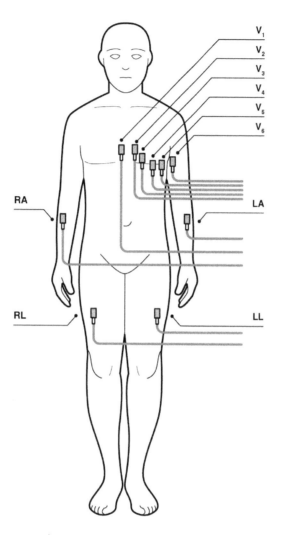

Patient Prep

In order to ensure an accurate tracing, the provider will:

- Explain the procedure to the patient.
- Expose the chest as necessary.
- Clip or shave excess hair as consistent with agency policy.
- Wipe the skin surface with gauze to decrease electrical resistance.
- Remove excess oils with alcohol wipe if necessary.
- Verify that the electrode is intact with sufficient gel.
- Attach the electrodes as appropriate.
- Complete the tracing.

Recognize Artifacts

Artifact is most often the result of patient movement while the tracing is being recorded, and the provider must be able to differentiate between the artifact and lethal arrhythmias. Artifact is most often evidenced by a chaotic wave pattern that interrupts a normal rhythm, as shown in the figure below.

EKG Artifact

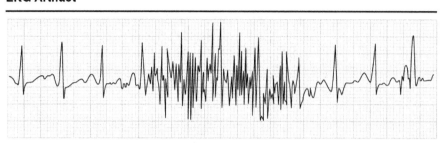

Recognize Rhythms, Arrhythmias

Normal Sinus: The rhythm originates in the sinoatrial (SA) node as indicated by the presence of an upright p wave in lead 2. A p wave precedes every QRS complex, and the rhythm is regular at sixty to one hundred beats per minute.

Normal Sinus Rhythm

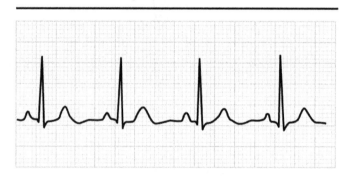

Sinus Tachycardia: The rhythm originates in the SA node as indicated by the presence of an upright p wave in lead 2. A p wave precedes every QRS complex, and the rhythm is regular at a rate greater than one hundred beats per minute.

Sinus Tachycardia

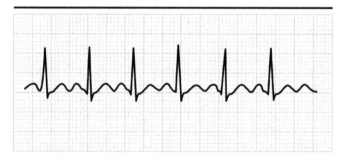

Sinus Bradycardia: The rhythm originates in the SA node as indicated by the presence of an upright p wave in lead 2. A p wave precedes every QRS complex, and the rhythm is regular at less than sixty beats per minute.

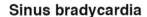

Sinus bradycardia

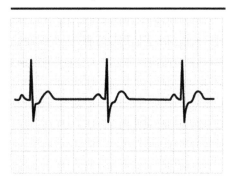

Atrial Fibrillation: The SA node fires chaotically at a rapid rate, while the ventricles contract at a slower but inefficient rate in response to an impulse from an alternative site in the heart. Individual p waves are not visible due to the rapid rate, and the QRS complexes are generally wider than the QRS complexes in the sinus rhythms.

Atrial Fibrillation

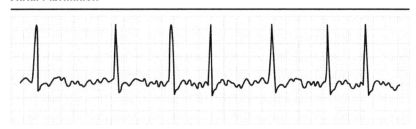

Complete Heart Block: The SA node generates a p wave that is not transmitted to the ventricles. The ventricles respond to an impulse from an alternative site, and the resulting complex has no association with the p wave. This condition requires immediate intervention.

Complete Heart Block

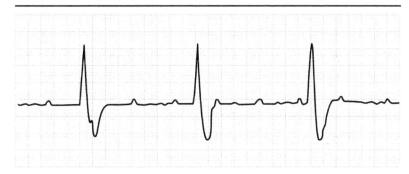

Ventricle Fibrillation: There is only erratic electrical activity resulting in quivering of the heart muscle. Immediate intervention is necessary.

Ventricular Fibrillation

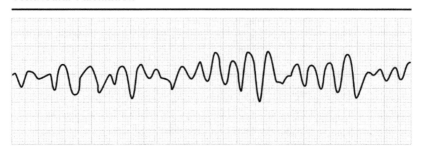

Rhythm Strips

The provider can use a six- to ten-second strip of cardiac activity to identify the heart rate and rhythm. The ECG paper is standardized to measure time from left to right, with each small box equal to four-tenths of a second, which means that each large box is equal to one-fifth of a second and the time elapsed between the black ticks is three seconds. The provider calculates the heart rate by dividing 300 by the number of large squares between two QRS complexes. In the figure below, the heart rate is 300/4 = 75. Alternatively, the provider can identify the heart rate by counting the number of QRS complexes in a ten-second EKG strip and multiplying that result by ten.

The provider will assess the rhythm by comparing the distance between complexes 1 and 2 with the distance between complexes 2 and 3.

Cardiac Rhythm Strip

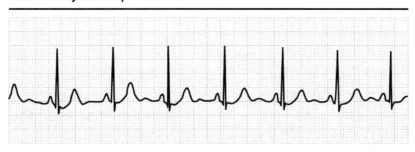

Holter Monitor
The Holter monitor is a portable device that is used for monitoring the EKG/ECG. The monitor may be used for routine cardiac monitoring or for diagnosing cardiac conditions that may not be evident on a single EKG/ECG tracing. The provider will attach the leads to the patient's chest, verify the patient's

understanding of the process, and provide the patient with a diary with instructions to record all activity and physical symptoms for the duration of the testing period.

Holter monitor with EKG reading

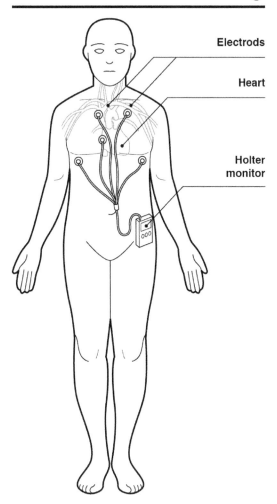

Cardiac Stress Test
The provider uses the cardiac stress test to identify the patient's cardiac response to the stress of exercise. The cardiac activity is recorded after the patient's heart rate reaches a target rate that is equal to 220 minus the patient's age. There are two forms of the test, which include the treadmill test and the pharmacologic test. Patients who are physically able walk on the treadmill until the target heart rate is achieved. Patients who are unable to tolerate the exercise will receive medications to raise the heart rate to the desired level. The provider will reverse the effects of these medications as soon as the appropriate tracings are obtained.

Vision Tests

Color
The most commonly used test for color blindness is the Ishihara Color Vision Test, which is a series of circular images that are composed of colored dots. The identification of the numbers embedded in the colored plates is determined by the patient's ability to identify the red/green numbers and background.

There are currently online variations of this test in addition to color testing forms that the provider may use for younger children who are not yet able to identify numbers.

Acuity/Distance

Snellen Chart

The chart contains eleven rows of letters that differ in size from row to row and is viewed from a distance of twenty feet. The resulting numbers, 20/100 for example, indicate that the patient can see objects at a distance of 20 feet that are visible to a person with normal eyesight at a distance of 100 feet.

E Chart

The E chart contains nine rows of letters that differ in size from row to row depicting the letter E is alternating positions. The chart is useful for children and others who are not familiar with the English alphabet. The scoring is similar to the Snellen chart.

Jaeger Card

The Jaeger card uses six paragraphs in differing font sizes ranging from 14 point to 3 point Times New Roman font to test near vision. The J1 paragraph at 3 point Times New Roman font is considered to equal 20/20 vision per the Snellen chart.

Ocular Pressure

The provider uses a tonometer to touch the surface of the patient's anesthetized cornea in order to record the pressure inside the eye.

Visual Fields

Visual fields are defined as the total horizontal and vertical range of vision when the patient's eye is centrally focused. The provider may use this test to detect "blind spots" or scotomas.

Audiometric/Hearing Tests

Pure-Tone Audiometry

The patient's pure-tone threshold is identified as the lowest decibel level at which sounds are heard 50 percent of the time.

Speech and Voice Recognition

The speech-awareness recognition (SAT), or speech-detection threshold (SDT), is defined as the lowest decibel level at which the patient can acknowledge the stimuli. The test utilizes spondees—two-syllable words that are spoken with equal stress on each syllable—as the stimuli for this test.

The speech-recognition threshold (SRT), or less commonly speech-reception threshold, measures the lowest decibel level at which the patient can recognize speech at least 50 percent of the time. This test also may be used to validate pure-tone threshold measurements, to determine the gain setting for a patient's hearing aid, or to provide a basis for suprathreshold word recognition testing.

Suprathreshold word recognition is used to assess the patient's ability to recognize and repeat one-syllable words that are presented at decibel levels that are consistent with social environments. Human-voice recordings are used to present the words, and the patient's responses are scored. The provider may use the results of this test to monitor the progression of a condition such as Meniere's disease, to identify improvement afforded by the use of hearing aids, or to isolate the part of the ear that is responsible for the deficit.

Tympanometry
The provider uses a tonometer to assess the integrity of the tympanic membrane (ear drum) and the function of the middle ear by introducing air and noise stimuli into the ear. The provider then assesses the resulting waveform and records the results.

Allergy Tests

Scratch Test
The provider applies a small amount of diluted allergen to a small wound created in the patient's skin in order to identify the specific allergens that elicit an allergic response in the patient. The allergist will select up to fifty different allergens for testing, which means that the provider will make fifty small incisions or scratches in the patient's skin arranged in a grid system to facilitate the interpretation and reporting of the test results. The provider will observe the patient closely for a minimum of fifteen minutes following the introduction of the allergen for the signs of an anaphylactic reaction, in addition to signs of a positive reaction. The provider will document all positive results that are evidenced by a reddened raised area that is pruritic.

Intradermal Skin Testing
The provider may use intradermal injections of the allergen to confirm negative scratch tests, or as the primary method of allergy testing. Using a 26- or 30-gauge needle, the provider will inject the allergen just below the surface of the skin. The provider must closely observe the patient and record results based on the appearance of raised, reddened wheals that are pruritic.

Respiratory Tests

Pulmonary Function Tests
Pulmonary function tests evaluate the two main functions of the pulmonary system: air exchange and oxygen transport. The specific tests measure the volume of the lungs, the amount of air that can be can be inhaled or exhaled at one time, and the rate at which that volume is exhaled. The tests are used to monitor the progression of chronic pulmonary disorders, including asthma, emphysema, chronic obstructive lung disease, and sarcoidosis.

Spirometry
Spirometry is one of the two methods used to measure pulmonary function. The provider attaches the mouthpiece to the spirometer and instructs the patient to form a tight seal around its edge. The provider will then demonstrate the breathing patterns that are necessary for successful evaluation of each of the pulmonary measurements. The spirometry device calculates each of the values based on the patient's efforts.

Peak Flow Rate
Peak flow rate is defined as the speed at which the patient can exhale. This measure is commonly used to evaluate pulmonary function in patients with asthma.

Tuberculosis Tests/Purified Protein Derivative Skin Tests
Tuberculosis tests/purified protein derivative (PPD) skin tests are screening tests for the presence of ***Mycobacterium tuberculosis. The provider will use a tuberculin (TB) syringe to inject 0.1 ml of tuberculin*** purified protein derivative, the TB antigen, into the interior portion of the forearm. The solution forms a small, round elevation or wheal that is visible on the skin surface. The patient must return to the agency for evaluation of the site between forty-eight and seventy-two hours after the injection. The provider will assess the site and document the size of any visible induration or

palpable swelling. The provider will not include any reddened areas in that measurement. The provider will refer all results that exceed 5 mm for additional testing and treatment.

Distinguish Between Normal/Abnormal Laboratory and Diagnostic Test Results

Laboratory testing results identify both the normal range for the test and the patient's results, and most often laboratory personnel add these results to the patient's electronic health record. In the event of critical results that require immediate intervention, such as a blood glucose level of 600 mg/dl, lab personnel will report critical results to the provider according to the standard laboratory protocol. The certified medical assistant (CMA) will report all values that are above or below the normal values for an individual test to the appropriate authority per agency protocol. The provider will recognize normal ranges for common laboratory tests.

Test	Normal Range
Fasting Glucose	70-99 mg/dL
Hgb A1c	4.3%-6.1%
Hgb	12-16 g/dL
WBC	4-11 K/µL
Potassium	3.5-5.1 mEq/dL
BUN	7-22 mg/dL
Calcium	8.6-10.5 mg/dL

The physician or other provider who evaluates a diagnostic test will report the results as his/her impression of the findings and recommendations for additional testing. These results are entered into the patient's EHR and sent to the patient's provider; however, the CMA must be aware of the patient-care implications of all testing results.

Pharmacology

Medications

Classes of Drugs
The provider is aware that prescription drugs are classified according to the chemical activity of the active elements or by the target disease. This means that antineoplastic medications are chemically active against cancer cells, while antidepressant medications are used to treat depression.

In addition, certain substances are also included in one of five schedules according to the potential for abuse under the Controlled Substances Act. The provider must be aware that Schedule I substances, such as LSD and peyote, do not have any medical application, are not safe for use even under medical supervision, and are noted to have great potential for abuse. Schedule II through Schedule V include substances based on the potential for psychological or physical dependence exerted by the individual substance. The provider is aware that Schedule II substances, such as oxycodone, have greater potential for abuse than Schedule V substances, such as Robitussin with codeine.

Drug Actions/Desired Effects
The provider understands that the efficacy of any medication is determined by how well the medication acts to produce the desired effects. This assessment includes a cost-benefit analysis, which measures

the adverse effects of the normal action of the medication against the resulting improvement in the patient's condition or disease status.

Adverse Reactions

The provider must differentiate between the side effects of a medication and an adverse reaction to that medication. Side effects, common to all therapeutic agents, are often temporary reactions to a given medication that seldom require   intervention or alterations in the medication administration. In contrast, adverse reactions are more serious events that often require the provider's intervention and discontinuation of the therapy. Adverse reactions can result from an allergic reaction to the medication, an exaggerated response to the drug action, or provider error, and the provider must document and report all of these events according to agency policy.

Physicians' Desk Reference (PDR)

The PDR is a directory of all prescription medications intended for the professional provider that includes all of the information contained in the package inserts provided by the manufacturer. The pharmaceutical companies publish annual updates of the PDR, which is also available as a consumer edition.

Storage of Drugs

The provider will meet safety and environmental requirements for all medications. All medications, including those that require refrigeration, must be secured in locked devices or medication areas. In addition, the provider will verify that the refrigerator is used exclusively for medication.

Preparing and Administering Oral and Parenteral Medications

Dosage
Metric Conversion
The provider must be able to calculate metric conversions as necessary for safe medication administration.

Units of Measurements
The provider will recognize common metric and household measurements, including liter, centimeter, milliliter, kilogram, gram, milligram, pound, ounces, tablespoon, teaspoon, foot, and inch.

Calculations
The licensed provider will calculate all dosage amounts with 100 percent accuracy according to agency protocol. Recent research indicates that the use of dimensional analysis to calculate intravenous (IV) drip rates and other dosage calculations is associated with improved provider accuracy.

Routes of Administration
The provider will utilize the appropriate administration route to ensure the optimum efficiency of the medication.

Intramuscular
The provider will use an intramuscular injection to ensure rapid absorption of a medication into the bloodstream when the intravenous infusion of the medication is inappropriate or inaccessible. Common sites for intramuscular injection include the deltoid, vastus lateralis, and ventral gluteal muscles.

Z-Tract Injection

When injecting medications capable of causing skin irritation or discoloration in the event of leakage from the injection site, the provider will apply traction to the skin surrounding the injection site with the nondominant hand, insert the needle into the muscle at a 90-degree angle, inject the medication, withdraw the needle, and release the traction on the skin, trapping the injected solution in the muscle.

Subcutaneous Injection

The provider will choose a subcutaneous site to inject medications that will absorb more slowly because of the limited blood supply in the fatty subcutaneous space. Using the nondominant hand, the provider will pinch the skin, insert the needle at a 90-degree angle into the fatty layer just under the skin, inject the medication, and withdraw the needle.

Oral/Sublingual/Buccal

The provider understands that the oral, sublingual, and buccal administration routes are appropriate for agents that will be rapidly absorbed into the bloodstream through the mucous membrane of the gastrointestinal tract. In addition, the sublingual and buccal routes are appropriate if the patient is unable to swallow a medication, or when the medication would be poorly absorbed or inactivated in the stomach. The provider is aware that sublingual and buccal medications are provided in tablet, film, and spray forms.

The provider will assist the patient to swallow oral medications that will be processed in the stomach or small intestine.

The provider will place sublingual medications under the tongue to facilitate rapid absorption of the medication into the bloodstream.

The provider will place buccal medications between the cheek and the gum where the medication will be absorbed through the capillary bed.

Topical

Topical medications are applied to the skin, mucous membrane, or body tissue, and may be provided as transdermal patches; ointments, lotions, and creams; or powders. The provider will assess the administration site for local reaction, and will rotate the site as appropriate for transdermal patches. In addition, the provider will avoid personal contact with the medications that are commonly absorbed rapidly through the skin.

Inhalation

The provider understands that inhalant drugs are used to deliver the medication directly to the target organ, which results in more rapid and efficient local absorption of the medication, in addition to decreased systemic exposure to the effects of the medication.

The provider will use medication-specific metered dose inhalers, dry powder inhalers, or nebulizers to administer inhaled agents that may include antimicrobials and corticosteroids. The licensed provider is also responsible for verifying the patient's understanding of the proper use and administration of these medications.

Instillation (eye-ear-nose)

The provider understands that medications may be instilled into the eye, ear, or nose to promote absorption or to treat local irritation of the site.

To instill eye drops, the provider will clear any accumulated secretions, use the nondominant hand to expose the conjunctival sac, instill the prescribed solution into the inner canthus while avoiding any contact with the eye, and use a sterile cotton ball to dry the eyelid.

To instill eye ointment, the provider will clear any accumulated secretions, use the nondominant hand to expose the conjunctival sac, apply the prescribed ointment along the sac from the inner canthus to the outer canthus while avoiding any contact between the eye and the medication container, and use a sterile cotton ball to dry the eyelid.

To instill medications into the ear, the provider will warm the solution to normal body temperature, position the patient with the head turned to the unaffected side, gently pull the ear up and back, instill the medication avoiding contact between the medicine dropper and the ear canal, place a sterile cotton ball loosely in the outer ear and instruct the patient to remain supine for fifteen minutes.

To instill nasal drops, the provider will instruct the patient to gently blow his/her nose, position the patient supine with the head tilted back, and instill the drops while avoiding contact between the inner nares and the medicine dropper.

Intradermal
The provider will use a 1 milliliter tuberculin syringe with a 5/8 inch 25- to 27-gauge needle to inject the prescribed medication into the interior portion of the forearm. The provider must identify the appropriate injection angle for the prescribed treatment; for example, allergy testing requires that the injection is 15-to-20 degrees, while insulin may be injected intradermally at 90 degrees.

Transdermal
The provider understands that transdermal medications, which are absorbed through the skin, provide the continuous release of a precise amount of the medication for a specific period of time. When applying a new dose of the medication, the provider will remove remaining residue from the previous dose, verify that the skin is intact and free of irritation, and sign and date the patch. Birth control pills, smoking cessation medications, pain relief agents, and nitroglycerin are some of the medications that are applied transdermally.

Vaginal
The provider understands that vaginal medications, which are available as suppositories, foams, ointments, and sprays, are used to alter the pH of the vagina, treat local infection, and provide comfort. The provider will insert the suppository form into the vaginal vault where it will liquefy as a result of body temperature. The provider will apply the ointment and spray medications according to the manufacturers' directions.

Rectal
Antiemetics, analgesics, and cathartics are commonly available as suppositories. The provider will insert the rectal suppository above the internal anal sphincter to prevent displacement.

Injection Site
Site Selection
The provider will select the appropriate injection site with consideration of the age and stature of the patient and the administration requirements of the prescribed medication. The provider is aware that injection sites must be systematically rotated for medications such as insulin that are repeated daily.

Needle Length and Gauge

The provider will select the needle gauge and length that is consistent with the selected injection site and the administration requirements of the prescribed medication.

Medication Packaging

Multidose Vials

The provider will withdraw the calculated amount of medication from the multidose vial using aseptic technique to avoid contamination of the remaining solution.

Ampules

The provider will break the ampule using safety precautions related to glass breakage and withdraw the entire contents into the syringe. The provider will then verify that the syringe contains the calculated volume of medication, replace the needle, and administer the medication according to protocol.

Unit Dose

The provider is aware the patient's medications will most often be provided in single-dose amounts, as opposed to multidose amounts, in order to avoid medication errors.

Prefilled Cartridge-Needle Units

The provider is aware that injectable medications may be provided as prefilled cartridges with attached needles. Depending on the manufacturer, a nondisposable holder will be provided for the cartridge. The provider must verify that the prefilled cartridge contains the calculated dose.

Powder for Reconstitution

The provider will inject the prescribed amount of diluent into the vial, mix the solution, and withdraw the calculated amount of medication.

Six Rights of Medication Administration

The "six rights" must be addressed for every medication dose. The provider will:

- Use two means of identification (ID) to verify the right patient, which can include the patient's verbal report and the agency ID band.

- Verify the prescription and the medication as provided by the pharmacy.

- Compare the route of administration documented in the medication record with the original prescription.

- Verify the time schedule as documented in the medication record.

- Calculate the correct dose and verify the result with another provider as required by agency policy.

- Document the administration of the medication and the patient's response in the medication record according to agency policy.

Prescriptions

E-Prescribing

The licensed provider can use a secure computer network to send medication prescription orders to participating pharmacies as allowed by federal and state laws.

<u>Controlled Substance Guidelines</u>
The provider will understand that:

- Pharmacies require either a handwritten and signed prescription, a faxed copy of a handwritten and signed prescription, or a prescription transmitted on a secure computer network in order to dispense controlled substances.

- Individual state laws may impose limits on the number of times that a prescription for a controlled substance can be written for an individual patient.

- Prescription authority is granted to licensed providers in accordance with federal and state laws and professional practice acts in the individual states.

Medication Recordkeeping

The provider will meet all agency-specific requirements for data entry and error reporting in the EHR. The provider will correct errors on paper documents by drawing one line through the incorrect entry without obscuring the original text, entering the corrected information, and signing and dating the entry.

Immunizations

The provider understands that a vaccine for a specific disease will stimulate the patient's immune system to produce antibodies that will protect the patient against the occurrence or severity of that disease.

<u>Childhood</u>
The provider must be aware of current vaccination recommendations in children from birth to eighteen years of age for the following diseases: diphtheria, tetanus, pertussis (DPT); Haemophilus influenzae type B (HIB); hepatitis B; measles, mumps, rubella (MMR); pneumococcal infections; poliovirus; varicella; human papillomavirus (HPV); and meningococcal conjugate in adolescents.

<u>Adult</u>
The provider must be aware of current vaccination recommendations for adults that include initial and additional vaccination for the following diseases: diphtheria, tetanus, pertussis (DPT); pertussis (Tdap); Haemophilus influenza type B (HIB); hepatitis A and B; measles, mumps, rubella (MMR); pneumococcal infections, influenza, and herpes zoster.

<u>Recordkeeping</u>
Vaccine Information Statement
The Centers for Disease Control and Prevention (CDC) issues a Vaccine Information Statement that documents the benefits and risks associated with an individual vaccine.

The provider must supply the Vaccine Information Statement to the patient or the patient's legal representative before the vaccine is administered.

<u>Vaccine Storage</u>
The provider must meet all of the requirements for vaccine-specific storage as identified by the CDC. Specifications for storage temperature, preparation, inventory control, and transport are included in the CDC Vaccine Toolkit.

Emergency Management/Basic First Aid

Assessment and Screening

Treatment Algorithms/Flow Charts
The provider is aware that treatment algorithms provide a picture of the sequence of best practices for a disease, which includes decision alternatives relevant to the patient's responses. The provider will use a flow chart to identify the human and system resources necessary to provide care.

Triage Algorithms/Flow Charts
The provider must be aware that a triage algorithm prioritizes emergency treatment in the event of mass causalities. The START model is the most commonly used treatment algorithm that classifies patients according to an initial assessment of their condition relevant to the need for immediate or delayed intervention.

The triage flow chart identifies all of the resources required to address an emergency and can be used by communities and health care agencies to assess the emergency care systems.

Identification and Response to Emergencies

The provider will use basic first aid to respond to the following emergencies, and will access emergency care as appropriate.

Emergency	Basic First Aid Response
Bleeding/pressure points	Apply firm pressure to the site with a clean cloth
Burns (minor)	Rinse with cool water, apply aloe, cover with clean dressing
Cardiac and respiratory arrest	CPR (depending on training), activate emergency medical services (EMS)
Foreign body obstruction	Heimlich maneuver, back blows, abdominal thrusts
Choking	Heimlich maneuver, back blows, abdominal thrusts
Diabetic ketoacidosis	Recognize manifestations, activate EMS
Insulin shock	Recognize manifestations, offer candy if alert, activate EMS
Bone fractures	Treat bleeding, immobilize the limb, apply ice
Poisoning	Position on left side, identify substance, call 1-800-222-1222
Seizures	Position on side, protect the head
Shock	Elevate the feet, maintain body warmth, CPR as necessary
Cerebral vascular accident (CVA)	Recognize manifestations, activate EMS
Syncope	Elevate legs 12 inches; loosen restrictive clothing
Vertigo	Maintain safety, access care to treat the cause
Wounds	Control bleeding, cover with clean material, access emergency care (ER)
Cold exposure	Remove wet clothing, blankets for gradual warming, fluids if alert
Heat exposure	Activate EMS, cold packs to pulse points, cool environment
Joint dislocations	Immobilize the limb, apply ice, access ER care for dislocation
Asthmatic attack	Rescue meds, activate EMS if no improvement
Hyperventilation	Calm victim, use paper bag, activate EMS with c/o chest pain
Animal bite (minor)	Control bleeding, clean site, apply antibiotic ointment and cover
Insect bite	Remove stinger, assess for anaphylaxis, clean site and cover
Concussion	Activate EMS, assess breathing and level of consciousness

Office Emergency Readiness

Equipment
Crash Cart Supplies
The provider will verify that all supplies recommended for emergency resuscitation according to advanced cardiac life support protocols (ACLS) are available for use. The contents of the crash cart must be specific to the patient population (e.g., adult care unit supplies will differ from pediatric care unit supplies). In addition, the provider will verify that all sterile supplies have valid sterility dates.

Automated External Defibrillator (AED)
The provider will use the automated external defibrillator to recognize and treat lethal cardiac arrhythmias. The provider is also responsible for periodic testing of the AED function.

Emergency Response Plan
All health care agencies will create a plan that identifies the personnel, actions, and resources required to respond to any emergency. The provider will participate in the implementation of the plan as necessary. The provider will assist agency employees to implement the evacuation plan for all patients and staff.

Practice Questions

1. In what way does the skeletal system support the immune system?
    a. Bones support and protect the spleen
    b. Calcium is stored in the bones
    c. The bone marrow is the site of WBC production
    d. The osteoclasts make new bone cells when necessary

2. Which of the following is a change associated with the integumentary system in the elderly?
    a. Acne
    b. Psoriasis
    c. Vernix caseosa
    d. Collagen alterations

3. Which of the following is the best example of indirect contact?
    a. Shaking hands with a friend
    b. Children playing with blocks
    c. Sitting next to someone who is sneezing
    d. Caring for a patient with HIV

4. Which of the following is an example of objective data?
    a. EKG tracings
    b. Chief complaint
    c. Family history
    d. Present illness

5. Which of the following conditions is considered as an obstructive disorder of the respiratory system?
    a. Pneumonia
    b. Small cell cancer
    c. Emphysema
    d. Asthma

6. The medical assistant must report which of the following findings to the primary nurse immediately?
    a. Five-year-old boy, T=100.2 rectally, Heart Rate = 90, Respiratory Rate = 28, BP = 90/50
    b. Twelve-year-old girl, T=99.6 orally, Heart Rate = 110, Respiratory Rate = 30, BP = 150/92
    c. Newborn, T= 98.3 axillary, Heart Rate = 146, Respiratory Rate = 42, BP = 64/40
    d. Thirty-eight-year-old woman, T= 99.0 orally, Heart Rate = 72, Respiratory Rate = 18, BP = 120/78

7. Which of the following statements correctly defines the difference between sanitization and disinfection?
    a. Sanitization is the removal of all pathogens on inanimate objects
    b. Disinfection is more effective than sterilization for cleaning surgical instruments
    c. Sanitization inhibits the action of microorganisms
    d. Disinfectants can remove all pathogens from a surface

8. The CMA observes the following rhythm on the patient's cardiac monitor. Which of the following is the CMA's best response?

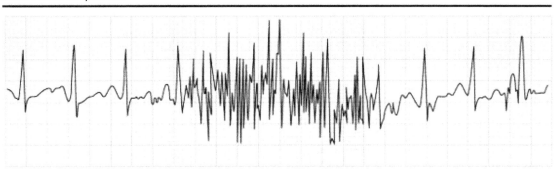

    a. Check the patient's electrodes to reduce the artifact
    b. No action is necessary because the tracing has returned to normal sinus rhythm
    c. Adjust the gain on the cardiac monitor to improve the quality of the tracing
    d. Notify the charge nurse and check the patient's vital signs

9. Which of the following identifies the correct procedure for collecting a twenty-four-hour urine specimen?
    a. For twenty-four hours, collect each individual urine sample, label the specimen, and transport it to the lab
    b. Discard the first voided sample, collect all urine voided for the subsequent twenty-four-hour period
    c. Collect and refrigerate all voided urine for twenty-four hours
    d. Insert an indwelling catheter to collect a sterile urine sample for the twenty-four-hour test

10. What is the difference between hemoglobin A1c lab test and the blood glucose test?
    a. The hemoglobin A1c lab test is a fasting test
    b. The blood glucose test must be drawn before breakfast
    c. The hemoglobin A1c lab test provides a three-month average glucose level
    d. The blood glucose test requires a venipuncture

11. The provider is conducting a physical urinalysis. Which of the following characteristics will be assessed?
    a. Turbidity
    b. Glucose
    c. Specific gravity
    d. pH

12. Which of the following characteristics is consistent with a diagnosis of bulimia?
    a. The disorder is common in men and women
    b. Refusal to consume any amount of food
    c. Damage to the oral cavity
    d. Long-term health effects are rare

13. The CMA is providing home care for a patient recently diagnosed with hypertension. Which of the following menu items is appropriate for this patient?
    a. Green salad with Ranch dressing
    b. Grilled cheese sandwich
    c. Grilled chicken and pasta
    d. Tomato soup and crackers

14. What is the main purpose of the Z-tract intramuscular injection technique?
    a. Identify patient-specific allergens
    b. Avoid possible local skin reaction
    c. Maximize the absorption of the medication
    d. Minimize the pain associated with the injection

15. The CMA will immediately report which of the following lab results?
    a. Hemoglobin A1c 6.2%
    b. BUN 19 mg/dl
    c. Potassium 2.8 mEq/L
    d. WBC 9,000 K/μL

16. The CMA is aware that an elevated C-reactive protein level is associated with which of the following conditions?
    a. Coronary artery disease
    b. Gastrointestinal bleeding
    c. Antibiotic sensitivity
    d. Pregnancy

17. What is dimensional analysis?
    a. A mathematical equation used to identify Body Mass Index (BMI)
    b. A process that uses three-dimensional positron emission technology (PET) scans to identify tumors in the body
    c. The automated cell counting process used to determine the WBC
    d. The process used to calculate medication doses

18. The CMA is providing home care for a patient who recently had a TB skin test. Which remark by the patient should be reported to the CMA's supervisor?
    a. "I will let the clinic nurse know when the spot turns red."
    b. "If the test is positive, I will need to take medication to treat the infection."
    c. "I should avoid people that have the flu."
    d. "If I have TB, my family will need to be tested as well."

19. The CMA is assessing the fluid intake of an assigned patient. The patient states that she drank an 8-ounce container of milk for breakfast. Which of the following is the correct documentation of this intake?
    a. 8 ounces
    b. 0.3 L
    c. 1 cup
    d. 240 ml

20. The CMA is providing home care for a patient with heart disease and diabetes mellitus. Which of the following manifestations is associated with diabetic ketoacidosis?
    a. Shaking and tremors
    b. Sweating
    c. Fruity breath odor
    d. Anxiety and irritability

21. The CMA has recently completed an in-service presentation about patient safety measures. Which of the following statements by the CMA indicates the need for additional instruction related to patient safety?
    a. "I will leave the beds in the lowest position."
    b. "If a patient is having a seizure, I will insert a tongue depressor to maintain the airway."
    c. "I will check the patient's documentation for fall precautions."
    d. " I will notify environmental services of any fluid spills."

22. Which of the following defines pure-tone audiometry?
    a. Subjective measure of the hearing threshold
    b. Speech discrimination measure
    c. Otoacoustic emission test
    d. Auditory brainstem response

23. Which of the following exam/position pairs is stated incorrectly?
    a. Vaginal examination: lithotomy position
    b. Sigmoidoscopy: prone position
    c. Fleet's enema: lateral position
    d. EKG/ECG: Fowler's position

24. The CMA is caring for a patient with hypertension who takes Digoxin. Which of the following patient remarks should be reported to the charge nurse?
    a. "I don't buy processed foods."
    b. "I take St. John's Wort for my depression."
    c. "I cook my vegetables without salt."
    d. "I will tell my doctor if I feel lightheaded."

25. A patient had an IV infusing at 50 ml/hour, a heparin drip infusing at 8 ml/ hour, an enteral infusion at 30 ml/ hour, and 50 ml of D5W with Clindomycin IV every six hours. The Foley catheter was emptied three times—450 ml, 375 ml, and 525 ml—and the total wound drainage was 46 ml. Which of these would be correct documentation of the twenty-four-hour intake and output?
    a. Intake = 2,312 ml, Output = 1,396 ml
    b. Intake = 1,920 ml, Output = 1,350 ml
    c. Intake = 1,520 ml, Output = 1,296 ml
    d. Intake = 2,200 ml, Output = 1,446 ml

26. Which of the following diseases is a vector-borne disease?
    a. Lyme disease
    b. Legionnaire's disease
    c. Varicella
    d. Impetigo

27. What are the manifestations associated with a serum potassium level of 7.5 mEq/L?
    a. This value is within normal limits.
    b. Anorexia and shortened Q-T interval on the ECG
    c. Paresthesias, elevated T waves and QRS widening on the ECG
    d. Prolonged P-R interval and U waves on the ECG

28. What is a "sick day" plan?
    a. Hydration regulations for a patient with cardiac disease who is experiencing flu symptoms
    b. Insulin administration protocol for Type 1 diabetics with decreased intake due to illness
    c. Antihypertensive medication plan for dialysis patients with fluid volume alterations
    d. Fluid rescue plan for infants with severe gastrointestinal losses

29. The CMA is reviewing the details of the DEXA or bone density screening test with a patient who is menopausal. Which of the following statements is consistent with this screening test?
    a. The scan can also identify arthritic changes in the hip joint.
    b. Medications containing magnesium should not be taken for 24 hours prior to the exam.
    c. The scan does not provide a reliable assessment of bone density in men.
    d. Fasting for 6 to 8 hours prior to the exam is recommended.

30. The CMA is caring for an elderly patient who often asks that words be repeated but is able to watch TV with the sound set at a normal volume. Which of the following interventions is most appropriate to the care of this patient?
    a. The CMA should speak more loudly when addressing the patient.
    b. The CMA should arrange for an interpreter who is fluent in sign language.
    c. The CMA should refer the patient to an audiologist to be fitted for a hearing aid.
    d. THE CMA should maintain a normal volume, speak slowly, and allow the patient time to process the conversation.

31. The CMA is discussing the purpose of buccal and sublingual routes of medication administration with a patient. Which of the following patient statements indicates a need for additional information?
    a. Buccal medications have an additional component that allows for the decreased permeability of the gums and palate.
    b. Sublingual medications provide immediate release of the medication to the systemic circulation.
    c. Buccal medications are formulated to withstand the acid environment of the stomach.
    d. Sublingual medications may exert a local or a systemic effect.

32. Which of the following is an age-related change in the GI system?
    a. Dry mouth or xerostomia
    b. Increased contractions of the upper esophageal sphincter
    c. Increased risk of peptic ulcer disease
    d. Malnutrition

33. The patient asks the CMA to explain how glaucoma affects the eye. Which of the following statements is the CMA's best response?

a. "Excess fluid collects in the front of the eye, potentially causing pressure on the optic nerve in the back of the eye, which can result in vision loss."

b. "Nerve damage causes the loss of central vision."

c. "Cellular debris eventually causes the lens to become cloudy, which decreases visual acuity."

d. "Changes in the blood vessels due to hypertension and hyperglycemia can increase pressure on the retina, resulting in blindness."

34. The CMA understands that a Safety Data Sheet (SDS) is required for every individual hazardous material present in an agency. Which of the following items are noted on the SDS?

a. Storage location of the substance in the agency.

b. Identification of personnel allowed to use the substance

c. First-aid instructions for the home user

d. Identification of potential hazards related to the use of the substance

35. Which of the following measurements is one of the mensuration assessment parameters?

a. Range of motion of the shoulders and arms

b. Fundal height in a pregnant woman

c. Bowel sounds

d. Body symmetry

36. Which of the following is NOT included in the Post-Exposure care of a healthcare worker following occupational exposure to the HIV virus?

a. Post-exposure anti-viral therapy is contraindicated if the exposed person is pregnant.

b. HIV testing will be repeated at 6 weeks, 12 weeks, and 6 months at a minimum.

c. The exposed person should avoid blood or tissue donation, breastfeeding, or pregnancy for 6 to 12 weeks after exposure.

d. Renal and hepatic studies and a CBC will be done at baseline and repeated frequently.

37. Which of the following menu choices is the best source of fiber?

a. 1 cup of fresh strawberries

b. 2 pieces of whole wheat bread

c. 1 ounce dry roasted almonds

d. 1 cup of split pea soup

38. A patient tells the CMA that he is doing well with his recovery from an MI 3 weeks ago. Which of the following statements by this patient indicates the need for additional instruction?

a. "I'm walking 20 minutes every day."

b. "My blood pressure is well controlled by my new medication."

c. "I think the ginseng that I am taking is helping me to exercise easier."

d. "I've stopped using salt at the dinner table."

39. The CMA understands that the vacuum tubes used to collect blood samples are color coded in order to identify the additive that is required for specific laboratory tests. Which of the following tubes contains a coagulant that facilitates the clotting of the blood in preparation for plasma tests?
    a. Tiger top (red/black)
    b. Red top
    c. Purple top
    d. Light blue top

40. As a community health care provider, the CMA must be aware of the manifestations of possible substance/alcohol abuse in the agency population. While many of the manifestations are common to both forms of abuse, which of the following manifestations most likely indicates substance abuse as opposed to alcohol abuse?
    a. Depression
    b. Violent behavior
    c. Lack of interest in the family or activities
    d. Abrupt weight changes

41. Which of the following lab reports is consistent with acute renal failure?
    a. BUN 12 mg per dL
    b. Serum creatinine 5.4 mg per dL
    c. Glomerular filtration rate (GFR) 92 L/minute X 1.73^2
    d. Hemoglobin 14.5 mg per dL

42. Diabetic ketoacidosis and insulin shock are life-threatening emergencies. Which of the following manifestations is an indication of insulin shock?
    a. Diffuse abdominal pain
    b. Anorexia
    c. Nausea and vomiting
    d. Sweating and anxiety

43. The human anatomy is divided into geographical planes for the purpose of identifying structures. Which of the following definitions is correct?
    a. The sagittal plane is a horizontal line that divides the core of the body into the right and left sides.
    b. The caudal plane is a vertical line that divides the body into the right and left sides.
    c. The transverse plane is a horizontal line that divides the body into upper and lower sections.
    d. The coronal plane is a vertical line that divides the body into upper or superior and lower or inferior sections.

44. A patient asks the CMA to explain the Jaeger chart. Which of the following statements correctly describes this chart?
    a. A series of paragraphs of increasingly smaller text that tests near vision
    b. A panel of letters of different sizes that tests visual acuity
    c. Circles containing colored letters embedded in a background of another color to test for color blindness
    d. A grid square of straight lines to test for macular degeneration

45. The CMA understands that the Clinical Laboratory Improvement Amendments (CLIA), established by Centers for Disease Control (CDC), the Food and Drug Administration (FDA), and the Center for Medicare and Medicaid Services (CMS), provide for the use of at-home laboratory tests. Which of the following criteria is NOT consistent with these amendments as they relate to waived test kits for at-home use?

    a. Waived lab tests will not cause harm if used incorrectly.

    b. The testing kits for at-home use must be approved by the FDA.

    c. The tests must not produce false-positive or false-negative results.

    d. Providers who recommend the use of the kits will provide appropriate instruction for their use.

46. Which of the following conditions requires that all who have contact with the patient use a particulate respirator capable of filtering particles smaller than 5 microns?

    a. Diphtheria

    b. Tuberculosis

    c. Adenovirus

    d. C. difficile infection

47. A patient is to receive Valsartan 0.16 g by mouth one time. There are 80 mg tablets available. Which of the following is the correct dose?

    a. 0.5 tabs

    b. 1.5 tabs

    c. 1 tab

    d. 2 tabs

Answer Explanations

1. C: The red bone marrow is the active site for production of stem cells, which are converted to WBCs to combat infection. The system does protect the spleen, store calcium, and make new bone tissue; however, these activities are not associated with the function of the immune system. Therefore, Choices *A, B,* and *D* are incorrect.

2. D: The collagen loses elasticity over time, which results in wrinkling of the skin in old age. The development of acne is most often associated with adolescence, but it may also accompany hormonal alterations in adult women. Psoriasis is an autoimmune disease that first occurs between fifteen and thirty-five years of age, but may appear in children. Vernix caseosa is the protective substance that protects the skin of the fetus during the last trimester of pregnancy. After birth, it provides the newborn with antioxidant and heat-regulation benefits. Therefore, choices *A, B,* and *C* are incorrect.

3. B: Indirect contact occurs when a susceptible person comes in contact with an organism that is present on an inanimate object, such as a child's toy. Shaking hands is considered as one-to-one or direct contact, while sneezing could spread infection by droplet or direct contact depending on the circumstances. HIV is most commonly spread by the exchange of blood and body fluids through close physical contact; therefore, Choices *A, C,* and *D* are incorrect.

4. A: Objective data is information that is observed by the provider, while subjective data is the information that the patient contributes to the health record. The patient supplies the data related to the chief complaint, family history, and the details of the present illness; therefore, Choices *B, C,* and *D* are incorrect.

5. C: Emphysema results in the failure of the alveoli and trapping of air in the distal airways, with resulting obstruction to the flow of air. Pneumonia is an infective process that may include the accumulation of secretions in the larger airways; however, air is not trapped in the airways. Small cell cancer is a neoplastic disorder that will affect lung function depending upon the size and location of the malignancy. Asthma is an allergic response to environmental antigens that is manifested by the stricture or closure of the airways; therefore, Choices *A, B,* and *D* are incorrect.

6. B: The heart rate, respiratory rate, and blood pressure BP are all elevated above normal for a twelve-year-old child. The other choices demonstrate normal values for the specific patient. The newborn has the most rapid heart rate and respiratory rate, which gradually decrease as the child matures; therefore, Choices *A, C,* and *D* are incorrect.

7. C: Sanitization is the process of inactivating or inhibiting, but not eliminating pathogens from a surface such as surgical instruments. Disinfectants are required to remove 99.9 percent of the *specific* susceptible agents; for instance, solution A may be effective agent B and C, but not agent D. Therefore, the solution is not 100 percent effective in eliminating infective agents from a surface. Sterilization is more effective than disinfection because 100 percent of all infectious agents are removed from an object; therefore, Choices *A, B,* and *D* are incorrect.

8. D: The middle section of this tracing is an artifact; however, the underlying rhythm is atrial tachycardia at a rate of one-hundred-fifty beats per minute. Therefore, the charge nurse should be notified and the patient's vital signs should be recorded. The artifact in this tracing is caused by the patient's movement, not faulty electrodes; therefore, Choices *A* is incorrect. The underlying rhythm in this tracing is not normal sinus rhythm because the rate is greater than one hundred beats per minute;

therefore, Choice *B* is incorrect. Adjusting the gain on the monitor will increase the amplitude of the complexes; however, it will not eliminate the artifact. Therefore, Choice *C* is incorrect.

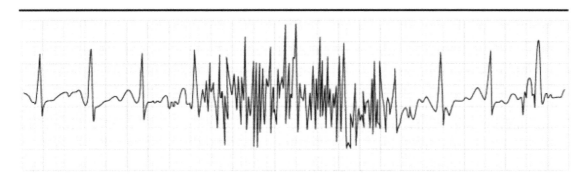

9. B: The first time the patient voids, the urine is discarded, and the twenty-four-hour testing period begins. This ensures that only the urine produced during the testing period is included in the analysis. The individual urine samples are collected in one container and are not submitted as individual specimens; therefore, Choice *A* is incorrect. The urine collection is usually refrigerated; however, the first voided sample must be discarded in order that only the urine produced during the twenty-four-hour test period is analyzed. Therefore, Choice *C* is incorrect. The twenty-four-hour urine collection does not require a sterile specimen; therefore, Choice *D* is incorrect.

10. C: The Hgb A1c test measures the percentage of the hemoglobin molecules that are "coated" or glycosylated with glucose. The hemoglobin molecule is a protein on the RBC, and the RBC has a lifespan of 120 days, therefore the resulting blood glucose value reflects the patient's blood sugar for the previous 120 days. The blood glucose test only measures the amount of glucose present in the blood at the time that the sample is obtained. The hemoglobin A1c lab test is a random sample that does not require fasting; therefore, Choice *A* is incorrect. The blood glucose sample may be drawn at any time. The fasting blood glucose level requires an eight-hour fast, and the two-hour postprandial blood sugar must be drawn precisely two hours after a meal; therefore, Choice *B* is incorrect. The blood glucose sample may be collected by finger-stick or venipuncture; therefore, Choice *D* is incorrect.

11. A: The physical urinalysis includes the assessment of the color and turbidity of the sample. Turbid urine is cloudy and, since freshly voided urine is normally clear, turbidity is an abnormal finding that may indicate the presence of other cells such as proteins or white blood cells in the urine. The provider uses reagent strips to conduct a chemical urinalysis that measures the glucose level, specific gravity, and pH of the urine sample; therefore, Choices *B, C,* and *D* are incorrect.

12. C: Bulimic patients consume large amounts of food in a short period of time, and then self-induce vomiting to prevent weight gain by disposing of the food. Stomach acids that are raised each time the patient vomits damage the mucous membrane of the mouth and the enamel layer of the teeth. Men and women are affected by eating disorders; however, more women than men are bulimic. Therefore, Choice *A* is incorrect. The bulimic patient consumes large amounts of food, but that intake is immediately followed by vomiting. The anorexic patient refuses to ingest any food; therefore, Choice *B* is incorrect. Eating disorders are difficult to treat and relapses are common, which means that long-term health effects are common. Effects can range from mild malnutrition to heart failure and death; therefore, Choice *D* is incorrect.

13. C: Hypertension is caused by narrowing of the blood vessels by fatty deposits, and is associated with fluid volume excess, which means that appropriate food choices should contain moderate amounts of animal fats and small amounts of sodium. Salad dressings, cheese, and canned soups all contain significant amounts of sodium and should be avoided; therefore, Choices A, B, and D are incorrect.

14. B: The Z-tract injection technique is used when the prescribed medication can potentially irritate or discolor the skin on contact. The retraction and release of the subcutaneous tissue decrease the possibility of any leakage of the medication onto the skin surface following the injection. Intradermal injections, not intramuscular injections, are used for allergy testing; therefore, Choice A is incorrect. Intramuscular injections are used to maximize absorption; however, the Z-tract technique is specifically designed to avoid skin irritation. Therefore, Choice C is incorrect. The Z-tract technique will not affect the pain associated with the intramuscular injection.

15. C: The CMA will immediately report the potassium level of 2.8 mEq/L, which requires intervention to avoid the development of cardiac arrhythmias. The hemoglobin A1c is minimally elevated, but this result does not require immediate intervention; therefore, Choice A is incorrect. Choices B and D are within normal limits and do not require intervention.

16. A: An elevated C-reactive protein level (CRP) is an indicator of the presence of an inflammatory process that has been identified as a risk factor for coronary artery disease. It also may indicate the presence of arthritis, pancreatitis, and kidney failure. The CRP is a serum test, not a stool test, which must be used to identify blood loss; therefore, Choice B is incorrect. Antibiotic sensitivity is identified by skin testing; therefore, Choice C is incorrect. Pregnancy tests measure the levels of human chorionic gonadotropin hormone, not the C-reactive protein; therefore, Choice D is incorrect.

17. D: Dimensional analysis is a mathematical process that is used to calculate intravenous and medication dosages. The research indicates that dimensional analysis results in fewer provider errors than the ratio and proportion calculation that is also commonly used in clinical practice. Dimensional analysis is not used in the calculation of the BMI. The equation for calculating BMI is indicated below; therefore, Choice A is incorrect.

$$BMI = \frac{Weight\ in\ Pounds}{(Height\ in\ inches\ x\ 2)}\ x\ 703$$

PET scans are imaging studies that use radioactive tracers to measure the chemical activity in the body, which is used to identify the presence of disease; therefore, Choice B is incorrect. The automated cell count devices use optical scanning technology to count body cells in the serum; therefore, Choice C is incorrect.

18. A: The TB test is evaluated by assessing the *wheal*, or indurated area at the site of the injection. Although a positive test may present as a reddened area surrounding the wheal, only the indurated area is measured and reported. The patient must return to the clinical agency for assessment of the results within forty-eight to seventy-two hours of the injection of the allergen, regardless of the presence or absence of redness at the site; therefore, the CMA must report the patient's remarks so that the licensed provider can reinforce the testing protocol. The remaining statements are appropriate and do not require intervention by the charge nurse; therefore, Choices B, C, and D are incorrect.

19. D: The metric system is used for all numerical documentation in the electronic health record, which means that the CMA will multiply 8 ounces times the conversion factor of thirty, which is the number of milliliters per ounce, to identify the appropriate number, 240 milliliters. Choices A and C are household measures and are therefore incorrect. Choice B is equal to 300 milliliters, which is more than the actual intake; therefore, Choice B is incorrect.

20. C: Fat will be used as an energy source when there is insufficient insulin to use glucose for energy production. If this condition exists for any extended period of time, the byproducts of the processed fats will accumulate in the blood. These ketones, or waste products, rapidly accumulate in the blood and the urine resulting in ketoacidosis. Small amounts of the ketones may be excreted with respiration as the lungs attempt to lower the levels in the circulating blood volume. This action results in the fruity odor of the exhaled air, which is a classic symptom of ketoacidosis. The remaining choices are manifestations of insulin shock, which are due to the effect of hypoglycemia on the nervous system; therefore, Choices *A, B,* and *D* are incorrect.

21. B: In the event of a seizure the provider will protect the patient's head from injury and assist the patient to the side-lying recovery position once the seizure is over; however, the insertion of tongue depressors is contraindicated because the oral cavity may be damaged, and there is clear research evidence that the patient's tongue will not obstruct the airway. The patient, especially the patient's head, should be protected from injury during the seizure; however, the provider should not restrain the patient in any way. The remaining choices demonstrate safe practice and do not require additional instruction; therefore, Choices *A, C,* and *D* are incorrect.

22. A: Pure-tone audiometry measures the patient's ability to hear tones at a certain decibel level. The results are compared to normal values to identify right/left deficits in the patient's hearing. It is a subjective test the patient signals when and if the tone is audible. The speech discrimination test measures the patient's ability to repeat words that are spoken through earphones at decibel levels consistent with hearing threshold levels that were previously identified; therefore, Choice *B* is incorrect. The otoacoustic emission test is an objective test that measures the response of the inner ear to a generated sound. This test is often used to assess hearing deficits in infants; therefore, Choice *C* is incorrect. The auditory brainstem response test measures the integrity of the neural pathway to and from the brain; therefore, Choice *D* is incorrect.

23. B: The patient is in the knee-chest position for a sigmoidoscopy in order to allow the insertion of the sigmoidoscope. The lithotomy position is appropriate for the vaginal examination, the lateral position is appropriate for the administration of the Fleet's enema, and the Fowler's position is appropriate for the EKG; therefore, Choices *A, C,* and *D* are correctly stated.

24. B: St. John's Wort may provide some improvement in depressive symptoms, but there is also evidence that regular use of the substance decreases the effectiveness of digoxin; therefore, the CMA should report this remark to the charge nurse. Limiting prepackaged foods and cooking without salt limits sodium intake, which is appropriate for a patient with hypertension. Recognizing that syncope is a possible side effect is also appropriate; therefore, Choices *A, C,* and *D* are incorrect.

25. A:

	Intake	Output
D5W 24 x 50 =	1,200	Urine = 1,350
Heparin 8 x 24 =	192	Wound = 46
D5W 50 x 4 =	200	
Tube Feeding 30 x 24=	720	
Total Intake	2,312 ml	Total Output = 1,396 ml

26. A: Humans contract Lyme disease by contact with deer ticks that are infected with the spirochete Borrelia burgdorferi. The causative agent is carried by the vector, the tick, that obtains the organism by a blood meal from the infected source, the deer, to the susceptible human causing the illness. Legionnaires disease is a severe form of pneumonia that is an airborne infection caused by the bacterium legionella. It was first identified in a hotel in Philadelphia where the infection was spread through the hotel's ventilation system; therefore, Choice B is incorrect. Varicella, chickenpox, is caused by the varicella zoster virus and can be spread through airborne, droplet, and contact exposure; therefore, Choice C is incorrect. Impetigo is caused by direct or indirect contact with objects that are contaminated with one of the causative organisms, Streptococcus pyogenes or Staphylococcus aureus; therefore, Choice D is incorrect.

27. C: The normal serum potassium level is 3.5 – 5.0 mEq/L. Elevated potassium levels are manifested by peripheral paresthesias and elevated, peaked T waves and increased impulse conduction time across the heart resulting in a widened QRS complex on the ECG. This value represents a severe elevation of the serum potassium level; therefore, Choice A is incorrect. Anorexia and a shortened Q-T interval on the ECG are associated with hypercalcemia, and elevated calcium level, therefore Choice B is incorrect. Prolonged P-R interval and the presence of U waves are alterations associated with hypokalemia, or a serum potassium level that is less than 3.5 mEq/L, therefore Choice D is incorrect.

28. B: Patients with type 1 diabetes have special needs for insulin dosage regulation depending on the specific illness. In general, patients are cautioned to not skip doses. However, the provider will identify a detailed plan for insulin administration and blood glucose monitoring for each patient. There may be patient-specific recommendations for the situations identified in the remaining choices. However, the "sick day" plan is most commonly identified with the care of the diabetic patient. Therefore, Choices A, C, and D are incorrect.

29. B: Although there may be agency-specific instructions, magnesium or calcium-containing medications are withheld to avoid interference with the scanned images. The scan is only able to identify bone density. Arthritic changes will not be visualized or evaluated. Therefore, Choice A is incorrect. Bone density testing is recommended for all at-risk populations including elderly men, therefore Choice C is incorrect. Fasting for this scan is not required or recommended, therefore Choice D is incorrect.

30. D: Current research indicates that many elderly individuals with normal hearing acuity may still have difficulty with conversation, especially in a noisy environment. The deficit is a delay in the processing or understanding the spoken word, not in "hearing" the words. The most useful strategy is to maintain a normal volume and allow extra time for the patient to process the words, therefore Choice A is incorrect. Sign language interpreters could only be helpful for a limited group of patients who might understand sign language, therefore Choice B is incorrect. Considering that the patient is able to watch TV set at a normal volume indicates that a hearing aid would not improve the patient's ability to process information, therefore Choice C is incorrect.

31 C: Buccal medications are absorbed at a predictable rate into the systemic circulation via the internal jugular vein, therefore the medication is not present in the stomach and will not be affected by the acid environment of the stomach. Because the palate and gums are less absorptive than the oral mucosa, the medications are formulated to provide predictable rates of absorption, therefore Choice A is incorrect. In contrast to buccal medications, sublingual medications that are surrounded by the oral mucosa are immediately absorbed into the systemic circulation, therefore Choice B is incorrect. Both sublingual and buccal medications can be used to exert local effects such as resolving mucosal ulcers, or for systemic effects such as the treatment of angina by nitroglycerin, therefore Choice D is incorrect.

32. C: With the normal aging process, the gastric mucosa loses some of the capability to protect against the formation of ulcers due to aging effects on the immune system, and when this process is associated with other existing comorbidities and NSAID use, the incidence of ulcer disease increases. Dry mouth is common in the elderly, but it is due to the effects of medication or disease, rather than the aging process, therefore Choice A is incorrect. The upper esophageal sphincter loses tone as a result of aging, which decreases the contractions and contributes to the incidence of gastric reflux, therefore Choice B is incorrect. Malnutrition is not a normal consequence of aging. It may be due to socioeconomic status or other personal issues; therefore, Choice D is incorrect.

33. A: Glaucoma occurs when the flow of fluid in the anterior portion of the eye is either slowed or blocked. The eventual change in the pressure in the eye can affect the optic nerve, which will lead to vision loss if the pressure is not controlled. The loss of central vision is due to macular degeneration, which is caused by injury to the macula, a small area on the retina that is responsible for maintaining sharp visional images, therefore Choice B is incorrect. Clouding of the lens is the defect associated with cataract formation, which is most often due to aging and is commonly treated by phacoemulsification surgery, which dissolves and removes the diseased lens and implants the new lens, therefore Choice C is incorrect. Diabetic retinopathy results from the effects of hypertension and increased blood glucose levels on the blood vessels in the retina, which result in swelling of the retina that causes abnormal transmission of impulses to the brain, therefore Choice D is incorrect.

34 D: The SDS includes potential hazards associated with the substance in order to protect employees from harm due to misuse. The SDS is issued by the manufacturer and will not contain any local information, therefore Choice A is incorrect. Agency policies regarding the use of hazardous substances may address personnel issues. However, the SDS strictly applies to the individual hazardous substances, therefore Choice B is incorrect. Consumer products containing potentially hazardous materials contain safety labels that may contain first-aid instructions, however the SDS is not required of consumer products, therefore Choice C is incorrect.

35. B: Mensuration is the process of measuring and includes parameters such as height and weight, and fundal height. Range of motion is assessed by the process of manipulation; therefore, Choice A is incorrect. Bowel sounds are assessed by the process of auscultation; therefore, Choice C is incorrect. Body symmetry is assessed by the process of inspection; therefore, Choice D is incorrect.

36. A: Anti-viral therapy will be started immediately after exposure, without waiting for further specialty consultation if the exposed person is pregnant due to the risk of the unborn fetus. HIV testing will be conducted at frequent intervals to monitor for the presence of evidence of infection, therefore Choice B is incorrect. The precautions listed in Choice C are necessary to prevent possible contamination in the event that the exposure has resulted in infection of the exposed individual by the HIV virus; therefore, Choice C is incorrect. Renal, hepatic, and hematology studies are monitored to assess any effects of the HIV virus and/or the effects of anti-viral medications if ordered; therefore, Choice D is incorrect.

37. D: One cup of split pea soup contains 4.8 g of fiber. One cup of strawberries contains 3 g of fiber, 2 pieces of whole wheat bread contain 3.8 g of fiber, and 1 ounce of dry roasted almonds contains 3 g of fiber.

38. C: Ginseng can potentially increase blood pressure and decrease the effectiveness of warfarin. Many over the counter preparations and herbal substances can alter the action of prescription medications. Therefore, patients should be encouraged to discuss all over-the-counter substances with their provider. Walking 20 minutes per day is an appropriate goal for this patient, therefore Choice A is incorrect.

Adequate blood pressure control and decreased use of salt are also essential to the patient's recovery from the MI, therefore Choices *B* and *D* are incorrect.

39. A: The tiger top (red/black) tube contains silica which promotes clotting of the blood to allow analysis of the clotting factors. The red top tube (glass) does not contain any additive and is commonly used for serological studies, therefore Choice *B* is incorrect. The purple top tube contains EDTA which is an anticoagulant, and this tube is commonly used for hematological studies, therefore Choice *C* is incorrect. The light blue tube also contains an anticoagulant, sodium citrate, which prepares the sample for Prothrombin time (PT), partial thromboplastin time (PTT), and fibrinogen studies, therefore Choice *D* is incorrect.

40. D: Abrupt weight loss or weight gain are common in individuals who abuse drugs because of the effect on the GI system and the brain. GI symptoms such as nausea, vomiting, and constipation may decrease food intake, while the "high" produced by the drugs produces overeating in some individuals. Individuals that abuse alcohol may become malnourished due to inappropriate food intake. However, the weight changes occur more slowly over time. Depression, potentially violent behavior and lack of interest in family and activities are common signs of both alcohol and drug abuse, therefore Choices *A*, *B*, and *C* are incorrect.

41. B: When the kidneys are damaged by disease or injury, waste products such as creatinine accumulate in the bloodstream, which means that a serum creatinine level of 5.4 (normal = .6 – 1.2 mg per dL) is a sensitive indicator of kidney function. The BUN level of 12 mg per dL is normal, and the CMA understands that the BUN is also affected by the patient's fluid volume status, which means that alterations in the BUN are not specific to kidney function. Therefore, Choice B is incorrect. The identified glomerular filtration rate in Choice *C* is also normal. Each of the stages of renal failure is defined by the GFR and the serum creatinine levels; therefore, Choice *C* is incorrect. Hemoglobin levels are decreased in chronic renal failure due to faulty erythropoietin regulation; however, the hemoglobin level in Choice *D* is normal; therefore Choice *D* is incorrect.

42. D: Insulin shock is a state of *hypoglycemia* and is manifested by sweating, anxiety, shakiness, and hunger. Diabetic ketoacidosis is a state of *hyperglycemia* and is manifested by malaise, weakness, fatigability, and GI symptoms that include abdominal pain, anorexia, nausea, and vomiting. Therefore, Choices *A, B,* and *C* are incorrect.

43. C: The transverse plane, also called an axial plane, is a horizontal line that divides the body into upper and lower sections. The sagittal plane is a vertical line, not a horizontal line, that divides the body into right and left sections, therefore Choice *A* is incorrect. Choice *B* is the definition of the sagittal plane, and since the caudal plane does not exist, Choice *B* is incorrect. Choice *D* is the definition of the transverse plane, not the coronal plane; therefore, Choice *D* is incorrect.

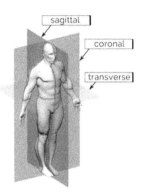

44. A: The Jaeger chart, used to assess near vision, is a card or sheet that contains a series of paragraphs that contain progressively smaller text. The Snellen chart is a panel with a series of letters of different sizes that tests visual acuity, therefore Choice *B* is incorrect. The Ishihara plates are used to identify color blindness by the identification of the colored number embedded in the circle, therefore Choice *C* is incorrect. The Amsler grid is a square with a grid of straight lines that is used to diagnose macular degeneration in the eye. If macular degeneration is present, the patient's view of the grid will be distorted; therefore, Choice *D* is incorrect.

45. C: The test kits must provide consistent results within a reasonable margin of error set by the FDA, which means that the potential for both false-positives and false-negatives does exist. Lab tests for home use are judged to be safe for consumers even if test is not used correctly, therefore Choice *A* is incorrect. All testing kits marketed for at-home use are approved by the FDA. Therefore, Choice *B* is incorrect. In order to optimize the validity of the results, providers who recommend the use of the at-home testing kits must provide the patient with appropriate testing instructions, therefore Choice *D* is incorrect.

46. B: Tuberculosis, varicella, herpes zoster, and rubella are transmitted by droplet infection, which means that all who come in contact with the patient must use a particulate respirator capable of filtering the infective molecules which are smaller than 5 microns. Diphtheria and Adenovirus are spread by droplet infection of causative agents that are larger than 5 microns, which means that a well-fitting surgical mask is adequate protection against contamination. Therefore, Choices *A* and *C* are incorrect. Contact precautions are required for the care of patients infected with ***Clostridium difficile*** (C-diff); however, masks of any type are not recommended, therefore Choice *D* is incorrect.

47. D:

$$Tabs: \frac{1\ tab}{80} \times \frac{1000\ mg}{1\ g} \times \frac{0.16\ g}{1} = 2\ tabs$$

Therefore, Choices *A, B,* and *C* are incorrect.

Dear CMA Test Taker,

We would like to start by thanking you for purchasing this study guide for your CMA exam. We hope that we exceeded your expectations.

Our goal in creating this study guide was to cover all of the topics that you will see on the test. We also strove to make our practice questions as similar as possible to what you will encounter on test day. With that being said, if you found something that you feel was not up to your standards, please send us an email and let us know.

We have study guides in a wide variety of fields. If you are looking for one, then try searching for it on Amazon or send us an email.

Thanks Again and Happy Testing!
Product Development Team
info@studyguideteam.com

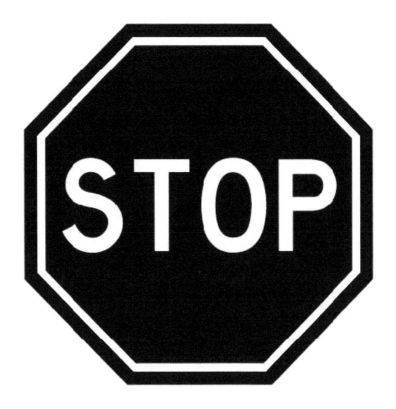

FREE Test Taking Tips DVD Offer

To help us better serve you, we have developed a Test Taking Tips DVD that we would like to give you for FREE. **This DVD covers world-class test taking tips that you can use to be even more successful when you are taking your test.**

All that we ask is that you email us your feedback about your study guide. Please let us know what you thought about it – whether that is good, bad or indifferent.

To get your **FREE Test Taking Tips DVD**, email freedvd@studyguideteam.com with "FREE DVD" in the subject line and the following information in the body of the email:

a. The title of your study guide.

b. Your product rating on a scale of 1-5, with 5 being the highest rating.

c. Your feedback about the study guide. What did you think of it?

d. Your full name and shipping address to send your free DVD.

If you have any questions or concerns, please don't hesitate to contact us at freedvd@studyguideteam.com.

Thanks again!

CPSIA information can be obtained
at www.ICGtesting.com
Printed in the USA
LVHW10s2300120918
590003LV00006B/82/P